Handbook of
Community Health Nursing

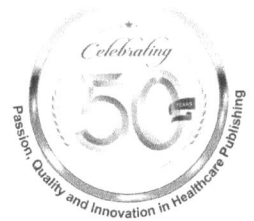

Handbook of
Community Health Nursing

Lakshmanan Mohan
MSc (Community Health Nursing)

Lecturer
Sitabai Nargundkar College of Nursing
Nagpur, Maharashtra, India

Foreword

S Kanchana

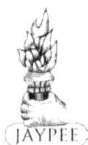

JAYPEE BROTHERS MEDICAL PUBLISHERS
The Health Sciences Publisher
New Delhi | London

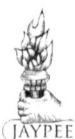 **Jaypee Brothers Medical Publishers (P) Ltd**

Headquarters
Jaypee Brothers Medical Publishers (P) Ltd
4838/24, Ansari Road, Daryaganj
New Delhi 110 002, India
Phone: +91-11-43574357
Fax: +91-11-43574314
Email: jaypee@jaypeebrothers.com

Overseas Office
J.P. Medical Ltd
83 Victoria Street, London
SW1H 0HW (UK)
Phone: +44 20 3170 8910
Fax: +44 (0)20 3008 6180
Email: info@jpmedpub.com

Website: www.jaypeebrothers.com
Website: www.jaypeedigital.com

© 2020, Jaypee Brothers Medical Publishers

The views and opinions expressed in this book are solely those of the original contributor(s)/author(s) and do not necessarily represent those of editor(s) of the book.

All rights reserved. No part of this publication may be reproduced, stored or transmitted in any form or by any means, electronic, mechanical, photocopying, recording or otherwise, without the prior permission in writing of the publishers.

All brand names and product names used in this book are trade names, service marks, trademarks or registered trademarks of their respective owners. The publisher is not associated with any product or vendor mentioned in this book.

Medical knowledge and practice change constantly. This book is designed to provide accurate, authoritative information about the subject matter in question. However, readers are advised to check the most current information available on procedures included and check information from the manufacturer of each product to be administered, to verify the recommended dose, formula, method and duration of administration, adverse effects and contraindications. It is the responsibility of the practitioner to take all appropriate safety precautions. Neither the publisher nor the author(s)/editor(s) assume any liability for any injury and/or damage to persons or property arising from or related to use of material in this book.

This book is sold on the understanding that the publisher is not engaged in providing professional medical services. If such advice or services are required, the services of a competent medical professional should be sought.

Every effort has been made where necessary to contact holders of copyright to obtain permission to reproduce copyright material. If any have been inadvertently overlooked, the publisher will be pleased to make the necessary arrangements at the first opportunity. The **CD/DVD-ROM** (if any) provided in the sealed envelope with this book is complimentary and free of cost. **Not meant for sale.**

Inquiries for bulk sales may be solicited at: jaypee@jaypeebrothers.com

Handbook of Community Health Nursing

First Edition: **2020**

ISBN: 978-93-89188-67-7

This book is dedicated with love and affection to my parents and to all community health nurses who have been the great source and inspiration and encouragement for me without whom this book would not have been completed.

Foreword

The *Handbook of Community Health Nursing* is written by Mr Lakshmanan Mohan, an alumni of Omayal Achi College of Nursing, Chennai, Tamil Nadu, India during his postgraduate program. One behalf of Omayal Achi College of Nursing family, I take pride in writing the foreword for his book.

At this juncture I wish to compliment, that the *Handbook of Community Health Nursing* adheres to the Indian Nursing Council (INC) syllabi and includes various assessments for all classifications, it gives an overview on Community Nursing diagnosis and also provides various checklist and formats to help the students utilize the same has a guideline during rural and urban community health nursing postings.

I congratulate Mr Lakshmanan Mohan, currently working as Lecturer at Sitabai Nargundkar College of Nursing, Nagpur, Maharashtra, India for making his dream a reality. I also pay my tribute to all those who have instrumental in motivating him to achieve his aspirations.

S Kanchana
Principal
Omayal Achi College of Nursing
Chennai, Tamil Nadu, India

Preface

Community health is an essential practice for achieving the goal "health for all". Health care has been for those who are not living near enough to a hospital and spend money for medicines and treatments. Majority of people stayed in rural area, where they suffer from health issues and even die without lack of care and medical facilities. To overcome this situation primary health care is basic care to reduce hospitalization and keeps the people healthy.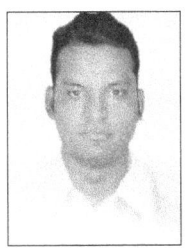

Being a community health nurse I strongly believe that health care will meet the health needs of the people by preventing minor ailments and providing primary care to reduce the morbidity and mortality of the people, its urged me to start working on this manuscript.

I hope this textbook would be useful for all Indian nursing fraternity.

Lakshmanan Mohan

Acknowledgments

I have put so much effort in completing this book. However, it would not have been possible without the kind support and guidance of many individuals and organizations. I would like to extend my sincere thanks to all of them.

My special thanks to my parents, friends, teachers, colleagues and students for the support and prayers which have made my dream come true.

Above all, I thank almighty God for being with me, guiding me and sustaining me in all my endeavors in completing this manuscript.

Contents

1. **Assessment of Various Age Groups-I**   1
   Newborn Assessment   1
   + Identification Profile   1
   + Anthropometric Measurement   1
   + Vital Signs   1
   + General Assessment   2
   + Role of Nurse   3
   Infant Physical Assessment   3
   + Identification Profile   3
   + Developmental Milestones   4
   + Anthropometric Measurement   4
   + Head to Foot Assessment   5
   + Systematic Assessment   5
   + Immunization   5
   + Inference   6
   + Role of Nurse   6
   Toddler Assessment   7
   + Identification Profile   7
   + Developmental Milestones   7
   + Anthropometric Measurement   7
   + Vital Signs   7
   + Head to Foot Assessment   7
   + Systematic Assessment   8
   + Immunization   8
   + Inference   8
   + Role of Nurse   8
   Pre-schooler Assessment   9
   + Identification Profile   9
   + Developmental Milestones   9
   + Anthropometric Measurement   10
   Infant and Children Protein-Energy Malnutrition Assessment   10
   + Early Detection and Referral of Children with Malnutrition   10
   + Vital Signs   10

- Head to Foot Assessment 11
- Inference 11
- Role of Nurse 12

School Going Assessment 12
- Identification Profile 12
- Developmental Milestones 12
- Anthropometric Measurement 13

Children Protein-Energy Malnutrition Assessment 13
- Early Detection and Referral of Children with Malnutrition 13
- Vital Signs 14
- Head to Foot Assessment 14
- Systematic Assessment 14
- Immunization 14
- Inference 15
- Role of Nurse 15

Adult Assessment 15
- Identification Profile 15
- Anthropometric Measurement 16
- Gomez Classification 16
- Vital Signs 16
- Head to Foot Assessment 16
- Systematic Assessment 17
- Inference 17

Antenatal History Format 17
- Demographic Profile 17
- Obstetric History 18
- Family History 19
- Medical-Surgical History 19
- Nutrition 19
- Partner's Health History 19
- Psychosocial History 20
- Antenatal Examination 20
- Head to Foot Examination 20

Intranatal Assessment Format 22
- Identification Data 22
- Present Obstetric History 23
- Antenatal History 23
- Past Obstetric History 23
- Physical Examination 23
- Vital Signs 24
- Mental Status 24

Contents **xv**

 Postnatal Assessment   26
 + History   26
 + Medical/Surgical History   27
 Nursing Care of Elderly in Emergencies   30
 + Assessment and Interventions to be Carried out in Emergency   30
 + Fluids   31
 + Aeration   32
 + Nutrition   32
 + Communication   32
 + Activity   33
 + Pain   34
 + Evaluation   34
 + Socialization   35
 + Mental Health   35

2. **Community Nutrition**   **37**
 Menu Planning   37
 + Explanation of Terms   37
 + Five Food Group System   39
 + Planning Diets   41
 Healthy Diet   51
 + Key Facts   51
 + Overview   51

3. **Minor Ailments and Home Remedies**   **55**
 + Household Cures   55

4. **Individual, Family, Community and Wellness Diagnoses**   **64**
 + Definitions   64

5. **Checklist**   **69**
 Checklist for Conducting Normal Delivery (Second Stage of Labor), Essential Newborn Care and Active Management of Third Stage of Labor   69
 Checklist for Newborn Resuscitation   77
 Checklist for Breastfeeding   78
 Checklist on Family Planning Counseling   79
 Checklist for Gestational Age Estimation   83
 Checklist for Administrating Injection $MgSO_4$ for Initial Management of Eclampsia   85
 Checklist for Management with Intravenous and Intramuscular Dose   86

*Checklist for Management of PPH due to
Retained Placenta 89
Checklist for Management of PPH due to Atonic Uterus 90
Checklist for Abdominal Examination 91
Checklist for Preparation of Labor Room 93
Checklist for Kangaroo Mother Care 95*

6. Formats 96
Community Survey Questionnaire 96
+ Part A: Socioeconomic and Demographic Profile 96
+ Part B: Village Profile 99
Family Case Study 99
+ Growth and Development 100
School Health Record 103

7. Procedure 105
Vaginal Examination 105
+ Checklist for Vaginal Examination during First Stage of Labor 105
BP Recording 106
+ Checklist for Blood Pressure Recording 106
Hb Estimation 107
+ Checklist for Hemoglobin Estimation 107
Urine Testing for Protein and Sugar 109
+ Checklist for Urine Testing 109
Bag Technique 110
Dementia Scale 113
+ Blessed Dementia Scale 113
+ Changes in Performance of Everyday Activities 113
+ Changes in Habits 113
+ Changes in Personality, Interest, Drive 114
Mini Mental Status Examination 115

8. Strategies to Control Emerging Diseases 116

9. Miscellaneous 122
+ Medical Abbreviation 123
+ Nursing Emergency Kit 124

Index 125

Introduction

Rapid social and economic growth in countries of the world has resulted in an increase both in the number of elderly people who are prone to degenerative and chronic diseases, and new patterns of illnesses that are brought on by social and economic factors such as occupational hazards, accidents, and environmental poisonings caused by air pollution, noise and contaminated water. Communities are struggling with a large number of people across the lifespan, who receive minimal or no health care because they cannot afford or access services. Moreover, public concerns regarding quality, cost, access and fragmentation of health care have contributed to a shift in care from the more traditional acute care settings to the community. This has led to changes in nursing practice. Nurses have always cared for individuals, families and communities in their practice. Recently, there has been an increase in the number of nurses working outside the hospital, primarily in community-based settings that focus on individuals and families. There is also increasing emphasis on community focused nursing care with the community as the client.

The population of ageing and chronically ill patients is increasing, and, coupled with the complex social conditions of today, has led to ill health, which increases hospital care expenses. Professional health services are not capable of meeting the ever-increasing demands of health care in this changing health culture. Evidence suggests that increasing attention to healthy lifestyles and healthy behaviors prevents health problems and reduces health risk and threats. Strengthening the community healthcare system based on primary health care is thus the focus of healthcare reform. Practically and preferably, professional nursing services focusing on providing health care and services to the entire community is an ideal solution to meeting the demands of community health care.

Definition

Public health is the Science and Art of:
- Preventing disease,
- Prolonging life,
- Promoting health and efficiency through organized community effort.

(Winslow, 1920)

Public Health is for:
- The sanitation of environment,
- The control of communicable infections,
- The education of the individual in personal hygiene,
- The organization of medical and nursing services for the early diagnosis and preventive treatment of disease, and
- The development of the social machinery to insure everyone a standard of living adequate for the maintenance of health.

1 Assessment of Various Age Groups-I

Newborn Assessment

IDENTIFICATION PROFILE

1. Name of the baby:
2. Age in days:
3. Gender:
4. Father's name:
5. Mother's name:
6. Place of delivery:
7. Full/pre-term:
8. Condition of birth:
9. Type of delivery:
10. Gestational age:

ANTHROPOMETRIC MEASUREMENT

1. Weight (kg):
2. Birth weight: Present weight [If weight is reduced more than 10% refer to Primary Health Center (PHC)]
3. Length (cm):
4. Head circumference (HC) (cm):
5. Chest circumference (CC) (cm):

VITAL SIGNS

- Temperature
- Heart rate (apical)
- Respiration
- Pulse

GENERAL ASSESSMENT

Assessment	
Activity	
Head	
Eyes	
Mouth	
Ears	
Nose	
Neck	
Chest	
Abdomen	
Umbilicus	
Genitalia	
Reflexes	
Moro	
Tonic neck	
Stepping	
Grasping	
Babinski	
Feeding Reflexes	
Rooting	
Sucking	
Swallowing	
Gag	
Protective Reflexes	
Blinking	
Cough and sneeze	
Yawn	
Urine	
Meconium	

Nursing Care

S. No.	Problem	Need	Nursing care

CONCLUSION

Common Problems

- Looks ill
- Poor breastfeeding or drinking
- Develop a fever or is cold to the touch
- Fast breathing

- Difficult breathing
- Blood in the stool.

ROLE OF NURSE

- Promote and support exclusive breastfeeding
- Advice the mother to maintain the hygiene of the baby
- Ask the mother to feed the baby every 2 hours.
- Teach the mother how to keep the young infant warm
- Teach the mother to recognize signs of illness for which to seek care
- Identify illness at visit and facilitate referral
- Give advice on cord care, hand washing and eye care
- Teach correct positioning of breastfeeding.

Good positioning is recognized by the following signs:	Poor positioning is recognized by any of the following signs:
• Baby neck is straight or bent slightly back, • Baby body is turned towards the mother, • Baby body is close to the mother, and • Baby whole body is supported	• Baby neck is twisted or bent forward, • Baby body is turned away from mother, • Baby's body is not close to mother, or • Only the baby's head and neck are supported

- Teach or educate about immunization.

Infant Physical Assessment

IDENTIFICATION PROFILE

1. Name of the infant:
2. Gender:
3. Father name:
4. Mother name:
5. Place of delivery:
6. Full/pre-term:
7. Date of birth:
8. Order of birth:
9. Condition at birth:
10. Type of delivery:
11. Medical history:
    - Past medical surgical history
    - Present medical surgical history
    - Family history
    - Personal history

DEVELOPMENTAL MILESTONES

S. No.	Milestones	Actual development	Child's development
1.	Cooing	3rd month	
2.	Social smile	5th month	
3.	Head control	6th month	
4.	Turned over	7th month	
5.	Crawling	9–10th month	
6.	Sits with support	9th month	
7.	Sits without support	10th month	
8.	Stand with support	10–11th month	
9.	Stand without support	11–12 month	

ANTHROPOMETRIC MEASUREMENT

1. Weight: Expected weight formula = $\dfrac{\text{Age in month} + 9}{2}$
2. Height (cm):
3. HC (cm):
4. CC (cm):
5. Vital signs
   - Temperature
   - Pulse
   - Respiration
   - Heart rate (apical).

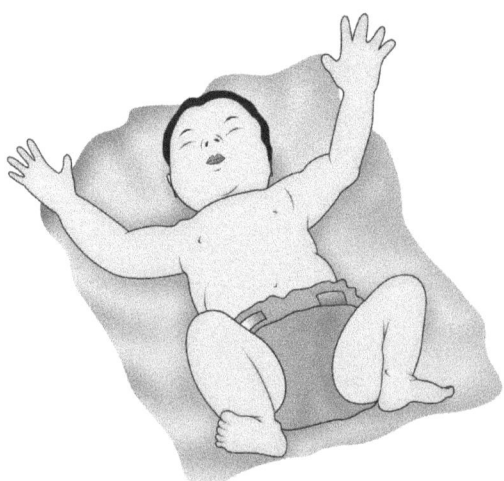

Fig. 1: Infant assessment.

HEAD TO FOOT ASSESSMENT

S. No.	Area	Findings	Inference

SYSTEMATIC ASSESSMENT

S. No.	System	Inspection	Palpation	Percussion	Auscultation

IMMUNIZATION

For Infants					
BCG	At birth or as early as possible till one year of age	0.1 mL (0.05 mL until 1 month age)	Intra-dermal	Left upper arm	
Hepatitis B - Birth dose	At birth or as early as possible within 24 hours	0.5 mL	Intra-muscular	Antero-lateral	
OPV-0	At birth or as early as possible within the first 15t days	2 drops	Oral	Oral	
OPV 1, 2, and 3	At 6 weeks, 10 weeks and 14 weeks (OPV can be given till 5 years of age)	2 drops	Oral	Oral	
Pentavalent 1, 2 and 3	At 6 weeks, 10 weeks and 14 weeks (can be given till one year of age)	0.5 mL	Intra-muscular	Antero-lateral side of mid-thigh	
Rotaviruse	At 6 weeks, 10 weeks (can be given till one year of age)	5 drops	Oral	Oral	
IPV	Two fractional dose at 6 and 14 weeks of age	0.1 mL	Intra-dermal two fractional dose	Intra-dermal: Right upper arm	

Contd...

Contd...

Measles/MR 1st dose	9 completed months-12 months, (can be given till 5 years of age)	0.5 mL	Sub-cutaneous	Right upper arm
JE-1	9 completed months-12 months	0.5 mL	Sub-cutaneous	Left upper arm
Vitamin A (1st dose)	At 9 completed months with measles Rubella	1 mL (1 lakh IU)	Oral	Oral

INFERENCE

Nursing Care

S. No.	Problem	Need	Nursing care

CONCLUSION

Common Problems

- Possible bacterial infection
- Jaundice
- Diarrhea
- Low grade fever
- Feeding problem or malnutrition
- Immunization status
- Other problems.

ROLE OF NURSE

- Promote and support exclusive breastfeeding
- Teach the mother how to keep the young infant warm
- Teach the mother to recognize signs of illness for which to seek care
- Identify illness at visit and facilitate referral
- Give advice on cord care and hand washing
- Teach correct positioning of breastfeeding
- Teach about immunization and then importance.

Toddler Assessment

IDENTIFICATION PROFILE

1. Name:
2. Gender:
3. Fathers name:
4. Mothers name:
5. Date of birth:
6. Order of birth:
   - Past medical surgical history
   - Present medical surgical history
   - Birth history:
   - Family history
   - Personal history

DEVELOPMENTAL MILESTONES

S. No.	Milestones	Actual development
1.	Throwing and kicking a ball (12 months)	
2.	Pushing and pulling (12 to 18 months)	
3.	Squatting (12 to 18 months)	
4.	Climbing (12 to 24 months)	
5.	Running (18 to 24 months)	
6.	Potty training (24 to 36 months)	
7.	Jumping (24 to 36 months)	
8.	Prereading (12 to 36 months)	
9.	Toilet training	

ANTHROPOMETRIC MEASUREMENT

Weight (Kg): Expected weight formula = Age in years × 2 + 8.

VITAL SIGNS

- Temperature
- Pulse
- Respiration.

HEAD TO FOOT ASSESSMENT

S. No.	Area	Findings	Inference

SYSTEMATIC ASSESSMENT

S. No.	System	Inspection	Palpation	Percussion	Auscultation

IMMUNIZATION

Completely immunized/partially immunized
If partially immunized why_____

INFERENCE

Nursing Care

S. No.	Problem	Need	Nursing care

CONCLUSION

Common Problems

- Upper respiratory tract infection
- Domestic accident
- Fungal infection
- Hook warm infestation
- Diarrhea
- Fever
- Malnutrition
- Other Problems

ROLE OF NURSE

- Provide cold compress to the child
- Dry the ear by wicking
- Assess the child feeding and counsel the mother accordingly
- Teach mother how to give oral drug and treat the local infections.
- Advise mother to give plenty of fluids to the child
- Teach her about the ORS therapy and its importance
- Teach about the personal hygiene to the child.

Chapter 1 Assessment of Various Age Groups-I

Pre-schooler Assessment

IDENTIFICATION PROFILE

1. Name:
2. Gender:
3. Father's name:
4. Mother's name:
5. Date of birth:
6. Order of birth:
7. Medical history:
   - Past medical surgical history
   - Present medical surgical history
   - Birth history:
   - Family history
   - Personal history

DEVELOPMENTAL MILESTONES

S. No.	Mile stones	Actual development	Child's development
1.	Physical growth	Weight: 16 kg Height: 80–100 cm Midarm circumference 13–16 cm	
2.	Motor development	Participate in sports activity	
3.	Gross motor development	Can throw balls skillfully over and underhand	
4.	Fine motor development	Build tower of 9–16	
5.	Self-care	Feeding skills: • Handless utensils skillfully • Enjoy eating selected stuffs	
6.	Sensory development	Visual activity is 20/20	
7.	Psycho-sexual	Latency period	
8.	Spiritual development	Mythic faith	
9.	Intellectual development	Concrete operational stage	
10.	Moral development	Conventional and pre-conventional	
11.	Language	Use more short sentences	
12.	Play stimulation	Jumping, group playing and rolls	

Handbook of Community Health Nursing

ANTHROPOMETRIC MEASUREMENT

1. Weight (kg): Expected weight formula = Age in years × 2 + 8
2. Height (cm): Expected weight formula = Age in years × 6 + 77
3. Mid-arm circumference (cm): 13–16 cm
4. Mid-upper arm circumference (cm): 13 cm.

Infant and Children Protein-Energy Malnutrition (PEM) Assessment

EARLY DETECTION AND REFERRAL OF CHILDREN WITH MALNUTRITION

Interpretation of Mid-Upper Arm Circumference (MUAC) Indicators

- MUAC less than 110 mm (11.0 cm), Red color, indicates severe acute malnutrition (SAM).
- MUAC of between 110 mm (11.0 cm) and 125 mm (12.5 cm), Red color (3-color Tape) or Orange color (4-color Tape), indicates moderate acute malnutrition (MAM).
- MUAC of between 125 mm (12.5 cm) and 135 mm (13.5 cm), Yellow color, indicates that the child is at risk for acute malnutrition and should be counseled and followed-up for growth promotion and monitoring (GPM).
- MUAC over 135 mm (13.5 cm), Green color, indicates that the child is well nourished.

Advantages of Mid-Upper Arm Circumference (MUAC) Screening

- It is simple and cheap.
- It is more sensitive.
- It is less prone to mistakes.
- It increases the link with the beneficiary community.

VITAL SIGNS

- Temperature
- Pulse
- Respiration.

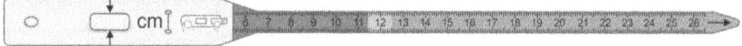

Fig. 2: Mid-upper arm circumference tape.

HEAD TO FOOT ASSESSMENT

S. No.	Area	Findings	Inference

Systematic Assessment

S. No.	System	Inspection	Palpation	Percussion	Auscultation

Immunization

Completely immunized/partially immunized
If partially immunized why_____

INFERENCE

Nursing Care

S. No.	Problem	Need	Nursing care

CONCLUSION

Common Problems

- Upper respiratory tract infection
- Domestic accident
- Anemia
- Fungal infection
- Hookworm infestation
- Diarrhea
- ENT problem
- Fever
- Malnutrition
- Other problems.

ROLE OF NURSE
- Provide cold compress to the child
- Dry the ear by wicking
- Assess the child feeding and counsel the mother accordingly
- Teach mother how to give oral drug and treat the local infections
- Advise mother to give plenty of fluids to the child
- Teach her about the ORS therapy and its importance
- Teach about the personal hygiene to the child.

School Going Assessment

IDENTIFICATION PROFILE
1. Name:
2. Age:
3. Gender:
4. Father's name:
5. Mother's name:
6. Date of birth:
7. Order of birth:
    - Past medical surgical history
    - Present medical surgical history
    - Birth history
    - Family history
    - Personal history

DEVELOPMENTAL MILESTONES

S. No.	Milestones	Actual development	Child's development
1.	Physical growth and biological	Weight: 22–32 kg Height: 121.5–136.5 cm Pulse: 85 ± 10 Respiration: 20 ± 3	
2.	Motor development	• Perform tricks on bicycle races • Throw balls • Use both hands independently	
3.	Self-care	• Feeding • Dress themselves and unaware of dirty cloths • Needs to remind brush teeth	

Contd...

Contd...

4.	Psychosocial	• Becoming peer oriented • Draws a person with 18–20 parts • Easy to get along with home • Has reasonable fear	
5.	Psychosexual	Latency stage (6–12 years)	
6.	Intellectual development	• Learns to understand and use abstracts symbols • Shows interest in casual relationship • Memory span increasing	
7.	Moral development	Conventional morality stage (need in law and order)	
8.	Language	Relative language, begin to use more compact sentences	
9.	Play stimulation	Prepare more companionship in play and enjoy making things	

ANTHROPOMETRIC MEASUREMENT

1. Weight (kg): Expected weight formula = $\dfrac{\text{Age in years} \times 7 - 5}{2}$
2. Height (cm):

Children Protein-Energy Malnutrition (PEM) Assessment

EARLY DETECTION AND REFERRAL OF CHILDREN WITH MALNUTRITION

Interpretation of Mid-Upper Arm Circumference (MUAC) Indicators

- MUAC less than 110 mm (11.0 cm), red color, indicates severe acute malnutrition (SAM).

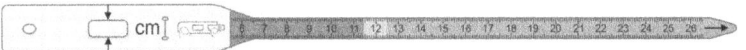

Fig. 3: Mid-upper arm circumference (MUAC) screening.

- MUAC of between 110 mm (11.0 cm) and 125 mm (12.5 cm), red color (3-color Tape) or orange color (4-color Tape), indicates moderate acute malnutrition (MAM).
- MUAC of between 125 mm (12.5 cm) and 135 mm (13.5 cm), yellow color, indicates that the child is at risk for acute malnutrition and should be counselled and followed-up for growth promotion and monitoring (GPM).
- MUAC over 135 mm (13.5 cm), Green color, indicates that the child is well nourished.

Advantages of Mid-Upper Arm Circumference (MUAC) Screening

- It is simple and cheap.
- It is more sensitive.
- It is less prone to mistakes.
- It increases the link with the beneficiary community.

VITAL SIGNS

- Temperature
- Pulse
- Respiration.

HEAD TO FOOT ASSESSMENT

S. No.	Area	Findings	Inference

SYSTEMATIC ASSESSMENT

S. No.	System	Inspection	Palpation	Percussion	Auscultation

IMMUNIZATION

Completely immunized/partially immunized
If partially immunized why_____

INFERENCE
Nursing Care

S. No.	Problem	Need	Nursing care

CONCLUSION
Common Problems

- Respiratory tract infection
- Anemia
- Viral infection
- Hookworm infestation
- Ear, nose, and throat (ENT) problem
- Fever
- Skin diseases
- Malnutrition
- Dental caries
- Vitamin deficiency
- Other problems.

ROLE OF NURSE

- Advice the child about personal hygiene
- Educate the child about dental caries and its prevention
- Assess the nutritional status and counsel the mother accordingly
- Teach mother how to give oral drug and treat the local infections
- Demonstrate about preparation of ORS for excessive dehydration
- Advice the mother to provide protein rich diet to the children
- Teach the child about oral hygiene
- Tepid sponge for the child with high temperature
- Check vital signs and observe the behavior changes.

Adult Assessment

IDENTIFICATION PROFILE

1. Name:
2. Age:
3. Gender:
4. Date of birth:

5. Address
   - Past medical surgical history
   - Present medical surgical history
   - Family history
   - Personal history
   - Nutritional assessment

ANTHROPOMETRIC MEASUREMENT
1. Height (cm):
2. Weight (kg): Expected weight formula = Height in cm −100 × 0.9
3. $\dfrac{\text{Actual weight}}{\text{Expected weight}} \times 100$

GOMEZ CLASSIFICATION

Gomez classification one of the earliest systems for classifying protein-energy malnutrition in children, based on percentage of expected weight for age.

Assessment of the Nutritional Status

Weight for age%	Malnutrition
91–100	Normal
76–89	1 degree
61–75	2 degree
Less than 60	3 degree

$$\text{BMI} = \frac{\text{(weight in kilograms)}}{\text{height in meters}^2}$$

VITAL SIGNS
- Temperature
- Pulse
- Respiration.

HEAD TO FOOT ASSESSMENT

S. No.	Area	Findings	Inference

SYSTEMATIC ASSESSMENT

S. No.	System	Inspection	Palpation	Percussion	Auscultation

INFERENCE
Nursing Care

S. No.	Problem	Need	Nursing care

Antenatal History Format

DEMOGRAPHIC PROFILE

Full name :
Age (in years) :
Education status :
Occupation :
Husband's name :
Age (in years) :
Education status :
Occupation :
Type of family :
Date of last antenatal visit :
Obstetric score
    Gravida
    Para
    Abortion
    MTP
    Living
Menstrual history:
Age at menarche
Duration of cycles

18 Handbook of Community Health Nursing

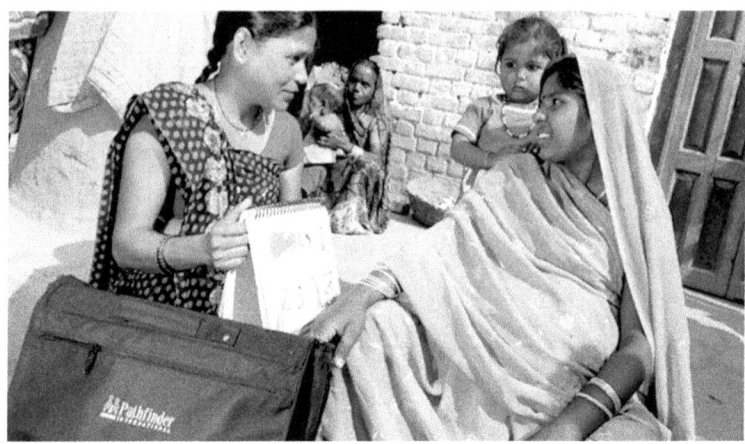

Fig. 4: Assessment in the rural community.

Regularity
Flow-Heavy/moderate scanty
 - Clots
 - No. of days
Any dysmenorrhea
  Relief measures
  Last menstrual period
  Estimated date of delivery (EDD)

OBSTETRIC HISTORY

Present Obstetric History

Is pregnancy confirmed?   Yes/No

When, where and how it was confirmed?

What test was done for confirmation?

Quickening

Immunization

Any more disorders like: Vomiting, hemorrhoids, heart burn, backache, bleeding, varicose vein, constipation, leg cramps, fever, leucorrhea, anorexia, insomnia, other complaints.

Past Obstetric History

No.	Year	Term/preterm/ stillbirth/ Live abortion	Type of delivery	If LSCS mention reason	Sex	Weight	Remarks

FAMILY HISTORY

- Congenital diseases
- Any hereditary diseases
- Multiple pregnancy
- Diabetes
- Heart disease
- Any mental retardation
- Hypertension or PIH (in mother/sisters)
- Twin pregnancy
- If yes,

In whom ? Mother/Father ?

MEDICAL-SURGICAL HISTORY

- Childhood disease
- Chronic disease like asthma, diabetes, epilepsy
- Previous surgery/ Lower segment cesarian section (LSCS)
- Injuries especially of back and pelvis
- Hepatitis, STD, HIV, Rh incompatibility
- History of anemia
- Any medication taken at present or past
- Reason for use, date stopped
- Blood transfusion, allergic reaction
- Any LSCS

NUTRITION

- General nutrition—veg/non-veg
- Appetite—decreased/increased
- Any eating disorders
- 24 hours recall

PARTNER'S HEALTH HISTORY

- Genetic abnormalities
- Chronic diseases
- Infections
- Use of drugs such as cocaine alcohol
- Smoking habits—tobacco, cigarette
- Sexually transmitted diseases—HIV/AIDS
- Blood type

PSYCHOSOCIAL HISTORY

- Emotional changes experienced
- Women's and family's reactions to present pregnancy
- Family support system—family members and friends
- Coping strategies
- Lifestyle change
- Social relationships with the neighbors
- Financial support

ANTENATAL EXAMINATION

General appearance :
Nourishment :
Body built :
Height :
Weight :
Vital signs : Temp
 : Pulse
 : Respiration
 : BP and SpO_2.
Mental status :

HEAD TO FOOT EXAMINATION

Skin turgor :
Moisture :
Warmth/temp :
Face :
Facial puffiness :
Lips : Cyanosis, dryness
Eyes :
Periorbital edema :

Chapter 1 Assessment of Various Age Groups-I

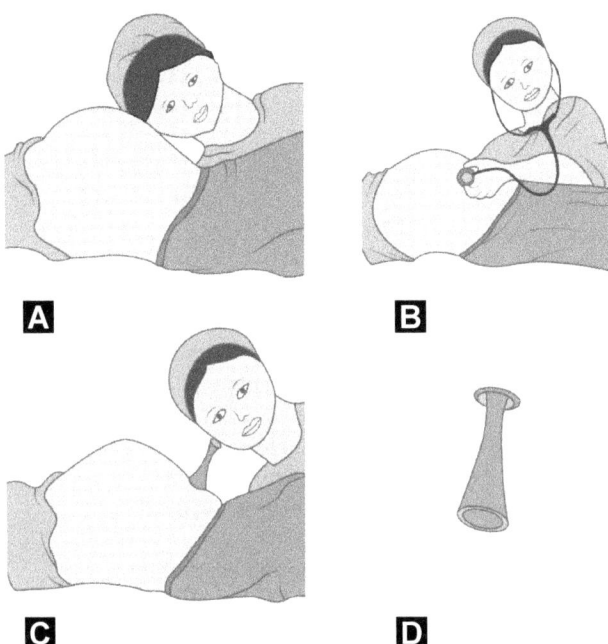

Figs. 5A to D: Antenatal assessment.

Conjunctiva	:	Pallor
Mouth	:	
Tongue	:	Moisture
Chest	:	
Thorax	:	Shape
	:	Symmetry of expansion
	:	Posture
Breath sounds	:	Vesicular sounds
	:	Wheezing/rhonchi
	:	Crepitations
	:	Pleural rub
Heart	:	Heart rate
	:	Location of apex beat/cardiac murmurs
Axilla	:	Any lymph node enlargement
Breast	:	Any tenderness/painful
	:	Tense/dilated veins/warmth/presence of crust/presence of montagometry tubercle
Nipples	:	Retracted/inverted/cracked

Abdomen   : Fundal height; Abdominal girth
Inspection   : Size, shape, contour, flanks, umbilicus, fetal movements, skin changes, contractions present/not, scars present/not, linea nigra present/not
Palpation   :
Fundal palpation   :
                           Inference : Lie
                           Presentation
Lateral Palpation   :
                           Left side : Description
                           Right side : Description
                           Inference : Position
Pelvic palpation   :
                           Pelvic grip : Description
                           Inference : Presentation
                           Engagement/not engaged
                           Attitude
                           Pawlick grip : Fixed/mobile
Auscultation   : FHR
                           Rhythm
                           Location
Extremities   : Ankle edema :
                           Capillary refill :
                           Cyanosis :
Vaginal Examination   :

Intranatal Assessment Format

IDENTIFICATION DATA
Name:
Age:
Education:
Occupation:
Husband's name:
Education:
Occupation:

PRESENT OBSTETRIC HISTORY

Last menstrual period (LMP):
Expected date of dilivery (EDD):
Period of gestation:
Gravida para living abortion (GPAL):

ANTENATAL HISTORY

- First trimester:
- Second trimester:
- Third trimester:

PAST OBSTETRIC HISTORY

Sl. No.	Dt./ Yr. of delivery	Place of birth	Duration of pregnancy	Method of delivery	Puerperium	Baby	
						Sex and weight	Present condition

Family history:

Medical/surgical history:

Personal history: Diet
  Rest
  Exercise
  Habits

Marital history: Consanguity/relationship

Socio-economic status:

PHYSICAL EXAMINATION

Nourishment:
Body built:
Height:
Weight:

VITAL SIGNS

Temp: - F/°C
Pulse: -/mt
Respiration: -/mt
BP -/mm of Hg.

MENTAL STATUS

Head to Foot Examination

Skin turgor:
Moisture
Warmth/temp:
Face: Facial puffiness:
    Lips: Cyanosis, dryness
    Eyes:
    Peri-orbital edema:
    Conjunctiva: Pallor
Mouth:
Tongue: Moisture
Abdomen
Inspection: Size, shape, contour, flanks, umbilicus, fetal movements, skin changes, contractions present/not:
Palpation:
Fundal palpation:
    Inference: Lie
    Presentation
Lateral palpation:
    Left side: Description
    Right side: Description
    Inference: Position
Pelvic palpation:
- Pelvic grip: Description
    Inference: Presentation
    Engagement/not engaged
    Attitude
- Pawlick grip: Fixed/mobile

Auscultation: - Fetal heart rate (FHR)
    - Rhythm
    - Location
Intranatal events: Time of onset of labor pain
Admission note: Maternal general condition
    Condition of uterus: Containing/not

Per vaginum (P/V) findings: Cervical dilation:
                             Effacement:
                             Station:
                             Membrane:
                             Liquor:
                             Pelvis:
Description of I stage:
Description of II stage:
Contractions monitored

Date	Time	Contractions			Fetal hear rate (FHR) (1 mt.)	BP (mm Hg)	Pulse (1 mt)
		Pregnancy	Duration	No. of contractions/ 10 minutes			

Per Vaginal Examination Findings

Date	Time	Dilation of cervix	Effacement	Station	Membrane	Liquor

Description of III stage:
Description of IV stage:
Condition of mother

    Condition of baby   *Placenta details*
    Weight: Weight:
    Cry: Cord length:
    Apgar score: Complete/incomplete:
    Vernix caseosa   Any abnormality of placenta
    Meconium aspiration
    Heart rate
    Any abnormality

Postnatal Assessment

HISTORY

Identification Data

Name:
Age:
Address:
Family income:
Occupation:
Date and time of delivery:
Place of delivery:

Present Obstetric History

- Parity
- Mode of delivery
- Normal vaginal
    - With episiotomy
    - Without episiotomy
    - With tear—first degree/second degree/third degree

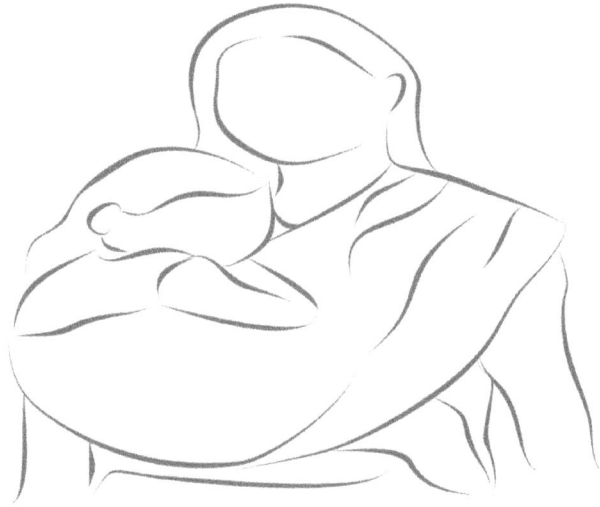

Fig. 6: Postnatal care.

- Spontaneous/medical/cesarean/any other
- Full term/premature
- Presentation (vertex/breech/shoulder/face)

Past Obstetric History

No.	Year	Term/preterm/stillbirth/live abortion	Method of delivery		Sex	Weight	Remarks
			Normal	ISCS			

Illness: TB/hypertension/diabetes/asthma/jaundice

MEDICAL/SURGICAL HISTORY

Any hospitalization
Surgeries
Medical condition

Family history: Illness-TB/hypertension/asthma/jaundice/diabetes

Medical surgical history: Any hospitalization
Surgeries
Medical condition

Personal history: Dietary
Habits
Use of contraceptives

Menstrual history

Psychological status: PPD

Physical examination

Nourishment   : Well nourished/undernourished
Body built   : Thin/obese
Activity   : Active/dull
Weight   : _____ kgs
Vital signs   : Temperature: _____ °C
Pulse   : _____ /mt
Respiration   : _____ /mt
Blood pressure   : _____ mm Hg
SpO_2

Mental status:
Consciousness : Conscious/unconscious/delirious
Mood : Anxious/worried/depressed.

Skin conditions
Color : Pallor/jaundice/cyanosis/flushing
Texture : Smooth/rough
Moisture : Moist/dry
Skin turgor : Hydrated/dehydrated
Temperature : Warmth/cold/clammy
Lesions : Macules/papules/vesicles/wounds
Presence of : Spider nevi
Palmar erythema
Superficial varicosities
Hyperpigmentation of : Areola nevi
Linea nigra
Chloasma

Head
Scalp : Cleanliness
Condition of the hair
Dandruff
Pediculosis
Face : Pale/flushed/puffiness/fatigue

Eyes
Eyebrows : Normal or absent
Eyelashes : Infection, sty
Eyelids : Edema/lesions
Eyeballs : Sunken/protruded
Conjunctiva : Pale/red/purulent discharge
Sclera : Jaundiced
Vision : Normal/shortsighted/longsighted

Ear
Hearing : Hearing acuity
: Any discharges/cerumen obstructing the ear passage

Nose
External hares : Crust ear discharge
Nostrils : Inflammation of the mucous membrane/septal deviations

Mouth and pharynx
Lips	: Redness/swelling/crusts/cyanosis/stomatitis
Odor	: Foul smelling
Teeth	: Discoloration/dental caries
Mucous membrane	: Ulceration/bleeding/swelling/pus formation and gums

Throat and pharynx : Enlarged tonsils/redness/pus

Neck
Lymph nodes	: Enlarged/palpable
Thyroid gland	: Enlarged

Chest
Thorax	: Shape
	: Symmetry of expansion
	: Posture

Breath sounds
	: Vesicular sounds
	: Wheezing/rhonchi
	: Crepitations
	: Pleural rub
Heart	: Heart rate
	: Location of apex beat
	: Cardiac murmurs
Axilla	: Any lymph node enlargement
Breast	: Secretion of colostrums /milk
Engorgement	: Any tenderness/painful
	: Tense/dilated veins/warmth/presence of crust
Nipples	: Retracted/inverted/cracked

Abdomen
Inspection	: Presence of scar/wound/fundal height
If cesarean	: Discharge/tenderness
	: Presence of striae
Palpation	: Height of the uterus: _____ cm
Consistency	: Hard/firm/boggy
Auscultation	: Bowel sounds _____ present/absent
Perineum	: Clean/Intact/tear/wound
Episiotomy	: Mediolateral/lateral/medial

Condition of the wound	: REEDA: Redness/edematous/ecchymosis/discharge/approximation

Lochia
i. Amount of bleeding	: Scanty/moderate/heavy
	: No. of beds changed _____
ii. Color	: Red/yellow/white rubra/serosa/alba
iii. Odor	: Fishy odor/foul smelling
iv. Clots	: Present/absent
Cervix	: Edematous/thin/fragile
OS	: open/closed
	: Any tear
Vaginal mucosa	: Smooth/distended/thin/atrophic
Vaginal introitus	: Erythematous/edematous
Bladder function	: Amount of urine output _____ mL
Bowel function	:
Hemorrhoids/anal varicosities	: Present/absent
Ankel edema/varicose veins	
Extremities	: Generalized muscular fatigue
Nails	: Color
	: Capillary refill
	: Shape

Nursing Care of Elderly in Emergencies

ASSESSMENT AND INTERVENTIONS TO BE CARRIED OUT IN EMERGENCY

F - Fluids
A - Aeration
N - Nutrition
C - Communications
A - Activity
P - Pain
E - Evaluation
S - Socialization
O - Others

Chapter 1 Assessment of Various Age Groups-I **31**

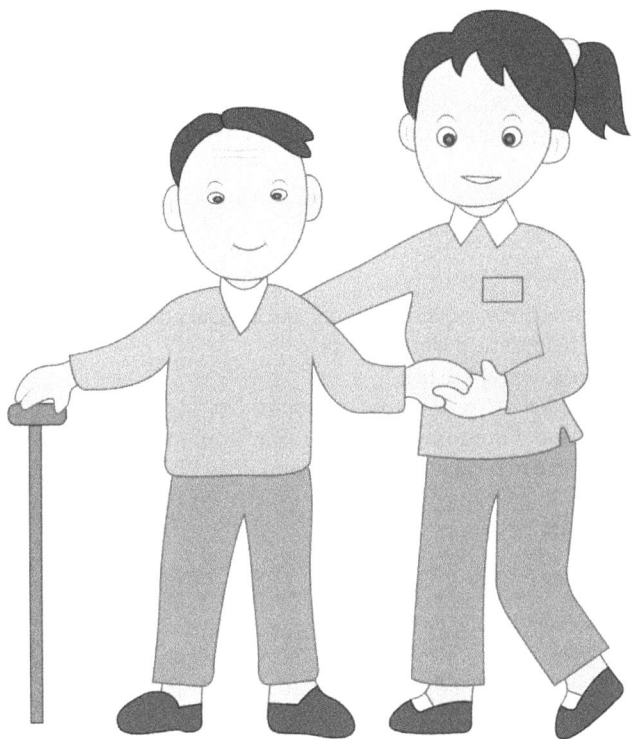

Fig. 7: Care of elderly.

FLUIDS

Assessment

Identify Person at Risk
- Geriatric with poor intake of water
- Dehydration
- Diarrhea and vomiting

Intervention
- Explain necessity of water intake and help water supply
- Provide medical treatment for dehydration as directed by the physician.

AERATION

Assessment

Assess the State of Ventilation (Adequacy of Oxygen)
- Overcrowded
- No. of windows and doors

Intervention
- Geriatrics can be separated and given special attention
- Keep the doors and windows open
- Use mosquito repellants
- Allow sunlight to pass across the room
- Garbages and dumping should be away from the shelter
- Toilets have to be kept disinfected and dry with deodorizing agents.

NUTRITION

Assessment
- Nutritional status
- Food intake
- Eating swallowing ability
- Use of dentures
- Toileting state
- Gastrointestinal symptoms

Interventions
- Ensure that food distributed is easily palatable (eat and swallow)
- High calorie food
- In case of malnutrition, determine weather admission to a hospital is required or not
- Seek for consultation with a dentist due to dentures and tooth defects
- Avoid foods such as:
  - Firm rice balls
  - Chilled packed lunch
  - Coconut fortified food as it can cause diarrhea
  - Dry brittle bread.

COMMUNICATION

Isolation in terms of information.

Chapter 1 Assessment of Various Age Groups-I

Assessment

- Voice quality
- Adequacy of teeth, tongue, larynx and pharynx
- Ability to read and understand spoken words.

Intervention

- Information said in a common site has to be interpreted as a brochures too.
- Transmission of information to the elderly has to be confirmed.
- Support should be provided for restoration procedures.
- Touch the elderly by pat to transmit information so as to give them a sense of well being.

ACTIVITY

Assessment

- Activities of daily living (ADL)
- Co-ordination
- Balance
- Strength
- Chronic illness
  - Diabetis mellitus (DM)
  - Hypertension (HT)
  - Coronary artery disease (CAD)
- Fracture or bruises
- Use of self help aids
  - Use of canes, walking stick or assisted walking devices
  - Use of spectacles.

Interventions

- Encourage activity
- Explain benefits of activities such as walking, exercise and promote them
- Relieve pain or swelling
- Help the diseased to continue with treatment and medication
- Prevent decrease in mental activity, i.e. encourage communication and be a good listener.

PAIN

Assessment

- Pain scale
  - Severity
- Characteristics
  - Intensity
  - Location
  - Duration of pain.
- American society for pain management nursing guidelines
  - Ask the patient about pain
  - Search for potential causes of pain
  - Observe behaviors
  - Seek surrogate reports of pain
  - Do an empiric analgesic trial.

Interventions

- Consider chronic conditions, especially musculoskeletal disorders and neuropathies.
- In the absence of self-report, observation of behavior is a valid approach to assess pain:
  - Guarding a body part, reluctance to move or be moved, decreased mobility, and crying out or wincing when touched.
- Fomentations can be given.
- Hot or cold applications can be given.
- Analgesics can be given as per order or standing orders can be implemented.

EVALUATION

Assessment

- Deterioration of health condition because of:
  - Insufficient intake of water and nutrition
  - Mental and physical fatigue caused by disaster
  - Poor living environment
  - Chronic diseases before the disaster

Intervention

- Secure and provide daily necessities:
  - Blankets
  - Warmers
  - Tatami mats

- Screens
- Drugs and wet compresses
• Evaluate and triage of elderly in need of support
  - Visiting health professionals
  - Volunteers
  - Long term care and welfare institutions
• Continue medication and diet therapy
• Provide information
  - Shelter pneumonia
  - Food poisoning
  - Economy class syndrome.

SOCIALIZATION

Assessment

- The degree of interaction
- Mobility
- Pre-disaster club activities
- Level of dependency

Intervention

- Make them participate in senior groups
- Learning new skills
  - Cards
  - Brain teasers
- Self help activities
- Encourage spirituality
- Organize games.

MENTAL HEALTH

Assessment

- Mental state
  - Anxiety/fretting
  - Irritation
  - Anger
  - Depressive tendency
- Sleep patterns
  - Insomnia
  - Feeling of sound sleep
  - Difficulty in falling asleep
  - Walking after the onset of sleep.

- Physical symptoms
  - Increase in blood pressure
  - Increase in glucose
- Living state and anxiety about the future
  - Living environment in the shelter
  - Personal relationships with surrounding people
- Symptoms of PTSD such as continuous crying when remembering the time of the disaster, insomnia and despondency.

Interventions

- Arrange assessment by health care practitioner and clarify the mental state of elderly evacuees
- Psychiatric consultation
- Identify aggravation of mental state
- When there are symptoms of PTSD, arrange for immediate visits to or by a psychiatrist or mental care specialist.

2
Community Nutrition

Menu Planning

Diet has a powerful yet complex effect on health. Dietetics is a science that deals with the adequacy of diets during normal life cycle and modifications required during diseased conditions. Menu planning is the process of planning and scheduling intake of meals for a general or specific individual requirements.

The following terms and concepts are widely used and a clear understanding of these terms makes Menu planning efficient.

EXPLANATION OF TERMS

Health is defined by the World Health Organisation of the United Nations as the "State of complete physical, mental and social well-being and not merely the absence of disease and infirmity."

The essential requisites (or dimensions) of "health" would include the following:
- Achievement of optimal growth and development, reflecting the full expression of one's genetic potential.
- Maintenance of the structural integrity and functional efficiency of body tissues necessary for an active and productive life.
- Mental well-being.
- Ability to withstand the inevitable process of ageing with minimal disability and functional impairment, and
- Ability to combat disease, such as
  - Resisting infections (immunocompetence)
  - Preventing the onset (and retarding the progress) of degenerative diseases such as cancer and
  - Resisting the effect of environmental toxins and pollutants.

Nutrient requirement can be defined as the minimum amount of the absorbed nutrient that is necessary for maintaining the normal physiological functions of the body.

Dietary reference intakes (DRI) values are replacing the traditional recommended dietary allowances in North America. This nutrient reference provides four sources of information:
1. *Recommended dietary allowances (RDA)*: The estimated nutrient allowance that is adequate in 97% to 98% of the healthy population specific for life-stage, age and gender. RDA includes addition of safety factor to the requirement of the nutrient, to cover the variation among individuals; losses during cooking and the lack of precision inherent in the estimated requirement. The RDA is the dietary intake goal for individuals, but its purpose is not to assess diets of individuals or groups.
2. *Estimated average requirements (EAR)*: The estimated nutrient requirement that is adequate in 50% of the population. This may be used to assess diets of individuals or groups, and is used to develop the RDAs.
3. *Adequate intakes (AI)*: Used when insufficient scientific evidence exists to calculate the EAR and RDA, and may be used as a goal for dietary intakes of individuals.
4. *Tolerable upper intake level (UL)*: The maximum nutrient intake that is not associated with adverse side effects in most individuals of a healthy population. This is not meant to be a recommended level of intake.

Nutraceuticals combine 'nutrition' and 'pharmaceuticals' to mean that food extracts can be used as preventive drugs or food supplements.

Functional food can be regarded as functional if it is satisfactorily demonstrated to affect beneficially one or more target functions of the body, beyond adequate nutritional effects. Functional foods must remain foods and they must demonstrate their effect in amounts that can normally be expected to be consumed in the diet. They are not pills or capsules but part of a normal food pattern.

Dietary/food supplements are concentrated sources of nutrients or other substances with a nutritional or physiological effect whose purpose is to supplement the normal diet.

Phytochemicals are of plant origin like terpenes, phytosterols, flavonoids, theols and allylic sulphides which are antimutagenic and anticarcinogenic agents and thus have nutraceutical properties.

Balanced diet is one which contains different types of foods in such quantities and proportions so that the need for calories, proteins, minerals, vitamins and other nutrients is adequately met and a small provision is made for extra nutrients to withstand short duration of leanness.

In addition a balanced diet should provide bioactive phytochemicals such as dietary fiber, antioxidants and other nutraceuticals which have positive health benefits. Low glycemic index food are preferred.

A balanced diet should provide around 60-70% of total calories from carbohydrate, 10-12% from protein and 20-25% of total calories from fat.

Balanced Diet

- Meets nutritional requirement
- Prevents degenerative diseases
- Improves longevity
- Prolongs productive life
- Improves immunity
- Increases endurance level
- Develops optimum cognitive ability
- Helps in coping up stress.

Thus balanced diet enhances quality of life.

FIVE FOOD GROUP SYSTEM

The five food group plan permits an individual to plan a menu to achieve nutrient intakes as specified by RDA. The five food group suggested by ICMR are given in **Table 1**.

The five food group system can be used by health professionals for the following purposes:
- *Tool for nutritional assessment and screenings*: A brief dietary history system can disclose inadequacies of nutrient from any of the five groups. The information can be the first clue for the possibility of the subject may be at the risk of developing nutritional deficiency.
- *Tool for nutritional counseling*: The dietary history based on the five food group system allows a health team to counsel or teach a patient about nutrition.
- *Explaining therapeutic diets to the patient*: Therapeutic diets are scientifically based on nutrient composition and groups which can be used in menu planning.
- *Food labeling and surveillance system*: Food groups can be used for food labeling and for nutrition surveillance system.

Food Exchange Lists

The exchange lists are the basis of a meal planning. Food exchange lists are groups of measured foods of the same calorific value and similar protein, fat and carbohydrate. All foods of exchange lists make a specific

Table 1: The five food groups and their major nutrients.

	Food group	Main nutrients
1.	*Cereal grains and products*: Rice, wheat ragi, bajra, maize, jowar, barley, rice flakes, wheat flour.	Energy, protein, invisible fat, vitamin B_1, vitamin B_2, folic acid, iron fiber.
2	*Pulse and legumes*: Bengal gram, black gram, green gram, red gram, lentil (whole as well as dals), cow pea, peas, rajmah, soyabeen beans.	Energy, protein, invisible fat, vitamin-B_1, vitamin-B_2, folic acid, calcium, iron, fiber
3	*Milk and meat products*: Mild, curd, skimmed milk, cheese, chicken, liver, fish, egg, meat.	Protein, fat, vitamin-B_2, calcium
4	*Fruits and vegetables*: *Fruits*: Mango, guava, tomato, papaya, orange, sweet lime, water melon. *Vegetables*: Green leafy—Amaranth, spinach, gogu, drumstick leaves, coriander leaves, fenugreek leaves. Other vegetables: Carrots, brinjal, ladies finger, beans capsicum, onion, drumstick, cauliflower.	Carotenoids, vitamin-C, fiber, invisible fat, vitamin-B2, folic acid, iron. Carotenoids, vitamin-B2, folic acid, calcium, iron fiber. Carotenoids, folic acid, calcium, fiber.
5.	*Fats and sugar* *Fats*: Butter, ghee, hydrogerated fat, cooking oils like groundnut, mustard, coconut. *Sugar*: Jaggery and sugar.	Energy, fat, essential fatty acids energy.

contribution to a good diet. None of the exchange groups can itself supply all the nutrients needed for a well-balanced diet. Exchange lists are based on principles of good nutrition that apply to everyone though extremely helpful for diabetics. Food exchange lists help in manipulation of protein, calories and other nutrients.

Food Composition Database

Food composition database are compilation of foods and their nutrient and non-nutrient components. All food groups are covered. The nutritive value is given per 100 g edible portion.

Energy content of food is calculated based on the content of protein, fat and carbohydrate.

Fat is measured as the fraction of the good soluble in lipid solvents which includes triacylglycerides.

Carbohydrate is a derived value obtained by subtracting the percentage of water, protein, fat, ash, crude fiber from 100 to give the percentage of carbohydrate 'by difference'.

Protein is measured as total nitrogen multiplied by a factor continues to dominate food composition. The general nitrogen conversion factor originally is 6.25 based on the assumption that protein contained 16% of nitrogen.

If data are not available, users with specific needs have two options:
- They can generate the data themselves, gathering representative sample of the foods.
- They can estimate impute the missing values from known data on similar foods and components.

National Institute of Nutrition

Indian Council of Medical Research, Hyderabad has published a book called 'Nutritive Value of Indian Foods'. The values given are average of many samples collected from different regions of India. One needs to keep this in mind while using these values.

PLANNING DIETS

People's eating habits vary enormously and dietitions must respect dietary freedom and diversity when making recommendations. Dietary diversity is one of our culture's strengths and sources of pleasure. There are many ways to eat to be healthy. The best way to achieve balanced diet is to plan meals in relation to other food for the whole day. It is advisable to eat small regular meals rather than one huge meal.

Principles of Planning Diets

- *Meeting nutritional requirement*: A good menu is one which will not only provide adequate calories, fat and proteins but also minerals, vitamins essential for the physical well-being of each member of a family. In a balanced diet the ratio of energy distribution from carbohydrate, protein and fat would be 7: 1 : 2. The diet should contain 'basic five food groups'.
- *Meal pattern must fulfill family needs*: A family meal should cater to the needs of the different members. A growing adolescent boy may need rich food to satisfy his appetite, whereas a young child may require soft and bland diet. Pregnant women require more greens in the diet. A heavy worker requires more calories and B vitamins than other member of the family. Meal pattern varies with age, occupation

and lifestyle of the family members. The family meal must offer children enough fat and flexibility in caloric density so that their energy needs are met.

- *Meal Planning should save time and energy*: Planning of meals should be done in such a way, that the recipes should be simple and nutritious. Labor and time saving devices can be used. Using convenience foods save time and energy.
- *Economic consideration*: Meals planned that are not within budget, cannot be put into practice. The cost of meals can be reduced by bulk purchasing and using seasonal fruits and vegetables.
- *Meal plan should give nutrients*: Losses of nutrients during processing, cooking should be minimized. Sprouted grams, malted cereals, fermented food enhance the nutritive value. Good quality protein should be distributed in all meals. Pressure cooker can be used to conserve the nutrients.
- *Consideration for individual likes and dislikes*: The meal planned should not only meet RDA but also individual preferences, particularly vegetarian or non-vegetarian preferences. If a person does not like particular greens, it can be tried in a different form or substituted by some other equally nourishing food. Food habits and dietary pattern should also be considered. Religion, traditions and customs of the individual should be considered in planning the menu.
- *Planned meals should provide variety*: If the meals are monotonous it is not consumed. Variety can be introduced in color, texture and taste, by using different kinds of foods and cooking methods. Variety also helps in meeting the nutritional requirement.
- *Meals should give satiety*: Each meal should have some amount of fat, protein and fiber to get satiety. Meals should be planned in such a way that interval between the meals is also considered.
- *Availability of foods*: Menus should include locally available foods. The wide variation in dietary patterns throughout the world depends largely upon the available food supply.
- *Health value of foods should be considered*: Ideal diets should provide besides nutrients those bioactive chemicals which can help to prevent and retard disease processes.

Following the international conference of Nutrition in 1992 the WHO and FAO recommended that all regions of the world provide advice to the public through qualitative and/or dietary guidelines relevant for different age group and lifestyles appropriate for the population. Food based dietary guidelines published as a technical bulletin by the WHO expresses the principles of nutrition education in terms of foods and reinforces the link between dietary pattern and reduced risk of certain diseases.

Points to be Considered in Planning a Diet

For a planning the menu the following points should be considered:
- For all nutrients minimum RDA must be met. For energy, the total calories can be RDA ± 50.
- Energy derived from cereals should not be more than 75 per cent.
- It is better to include two cereals in one meal like rice and wheat or millets and rice.
- Whole grain cereals, parboiled grains or malted grains give higher nutritive value.
- Flour should not be sieved for chapathi as it reduces bran content.
- Minimize refined cereals like maida.
- To improve the cereal and pulse protein quality minimum ratio of cereal protein to pulse protein should be 4:1. In terms of the grains it will be eight parts of cereals and one part of pulses.
- Two to three servings of pulses should be taken every day. Germinated pulses are more nutritious.
- One egg weighs around 40 g. This can be served along with cereal or pulses to improve the quality of protein. Instead, one serving of poultry/fish can also be included in the diet.
- A minimum quality of 500 mL milk/day should be included. Two glasses of milk or curd should be included in a balanced diet. Curd provides probiotics. Low fat milk should be preferred.
- Foods rich in fiber should be included in the diet.
- Every meal should contain at least one medium size fruit. It is better to serve the fruit raw. Taking juice out of it causes loss of vitamin C.
- Inclusion of salads or raita not only help in meeting the vitamin requirements but the meals would be attractive and have high satiety value due to the fiber content.
- Green leafy vegetables can be taken more than one serving. Colored vegetables and fruits are preferred.
- Five servings of colorful fruits and vegetables should be included in a day's diet to meet antioxidant requirement.
- Energy derived from fats or oils is 15–20 per cent of total calories and 5 per cent from sugar and jaggery.
- It is better to use more than one type of oil. Combination of oils have proper balance between n-3 and n-6 fatty acids.
- Choose a diet low in fat, saturated fat, trans fats and cholesterol.
- Fried foods cannot be planned if oil allowance is less or in low calorie diets.
- Variety of foods should be used in the menu. No single food has all the nutrients.
- Use salt and sugar in moderation.

- Ideally each meal should consist of all the five foods groups.
- Usually the number of meals would be four and for very young children and patients, number of meals can be more.
- One-third of nutritional requirement—at least calories and protein should be met by lunch as well as by dinner.
- For quick calculations food exchange list can be used.
- If possible, meals should be planned at a time for several days.
- Water should be taken in adequate quantities.
- Use processed and ready to eat foods judiciously. Processed foods contain a variety of food additives.
- Children and patients whose nutritional requirements are high, supplementary foods can be given.

Steps Involved in Planning a Diet

There are three steps involved in planning a menu:

Step I: Recommended dietary allowances

To calculate balanced diet, as a first step there is need to know recommended dietary allowances for different age groups prescribed by Nutrition expert committee of ICMR. **Table 2** shows recommended dietary allowances for Indians (1989).

Step II: Food List

Food list can be prepared either by using ICMR tables or exchange lists.

A. Using ICMR Tables

As a second step while planning the daily diet the foods are chosen from all five food groups. To make menu planning more convenient ICMR has suggested the portion size and balanced diets for adults and for different age group **(Tables 3 to 5)**.

The balanced diets for adults and different age groups are given as multiples of these portion sizes. The portion sizes are given in terms of raw food.

Quantity indicates top milk. For breastfed infants, 200 mL top milk is required one portion of pulse may be exchanged with one portion (50 g) of egg/meat chicken/fish.

B. Using Cooked Food Exchange Lists

The diet can also be prescribed in terms of exchange lists. Each exchange provides 100 kcal.

Table 2: Recommended Dietary allowances for Indians-1999.

Group	Particular	Body wt	Net energy	Protein	Fat	Calcium	Iron	Vitamin A		Thiamine	Riboflavin	Nicotinic acid	Pyridoxine	Ascorbic acid	Folic acid	Vit. B_{12}
								Retinol	β carotene							
		kg	kcal/d	g/d	g/d	mg/d	mg/d	µg/d	µg/d	mg/d	mg/d	mg/d	mg/d	mg/d	µg/d	µg
Men	Sedentary work	60	2425	60	20	400	28	600	2400	1.2	1.4	16	2.0	40	100	1
	Moderate work		2875						0	1.4	1.6	18				
	Heavy work		3800							1.6	1.9	21				
Women	Sedentary work	50	1875							0.9	1.1	12				
	Moderate work		2225	50	20	400	30	600	2400	1.1	1.3	14	2.0	40	100	1
	Heavy work		2925							1.2	1.5	16				
	Pregnant women		+300	+15	30	1000	38	600	2400	+0.2	+0.2	+2	2.5	40	400	1
	Lactation		+550	71	40	1200	30	1300		1.4	1.4					
	0–6 months		+550	+18	45	1000	30	950	3800	+0.3	+0.3	+4				
	6–12 months		+400	+18						+0.2	+0.2	+3	2.5	80	150	1.5
Infants	0–6 months	5.4	108/kg	2.05/kg						55µg/kg	65 µg/kg	710 µg/kg	0.1	25	25	0.2
	6–12 months	8.6	98/kg	1.65				350	1400	50 µg/kg	60 µg/kg	650 µg/kg	04			

Contd...

Contd...

Group	Particular	Body wt (kg)	Net energy (kcal/d)	Protein (g/d)	Fat (g/d)	Calcium (mg/d)	Iron (mg/d)	Vitamin A Retinol (µg/d)	Vitamin A β carotene (µg/d)	Thiamine (mg/d)	Riboflavin (mg/d)	Nicotinic acid (mg/d)	Pyridoxine (mg/d)	Ascorbic acid (mg/d)	Folic acid (µg/d)	Vit. B12 (µg/d)
Children	1–3 years	12.2	1240	22			12	400		0.6	0.7	8	0.9		30	
	4–6 years	19.0	1690	30	25	400	18	400	1600	0.9	1.0	11		40	40	02–1.0
	7–9 years	26.9	1950	41			26	600	2400	1.0	1.2	13	1.5		60	
Boys	10–12 years	35.4	2190	54			34			1.1	1.3	15	1.6	40	40	0.2–1.0
Girls	10–12 Years	31.5	1970	57	22	600	19	600	2400	1.0	1.2	13				
Boys	13–15 years	47.8	2450	70			41			1.2	1.5	16				
Girls	13–15 years	46.7	2060	65	22	600	28	600	2400	1.0	1.2	14	2.0	40	100	0.2–1.0
Boys	16–18 years	57.1	2640	78			50			1.3	1.6	17				
Girls	16–18 years	49.9	2060	63	22	500	30	600	2400	1.0	1.2	14	2.0	40	100	0.2–1.0

Chapter 2 Community Nutrition 47

Table 3: Portion size for menu plan.

Food group	Portion g	Energy kcal	Protein g	Carbohydrate g	Fat g
Cereals and millets	30	100	3.0	20	0.8
Pulses	30	100	6.0	15	0.7
Egg	50	85	7.0	–	7.0
Meat, chicken or fish	50	100	9	–	7.0
Milk	100	70	3.0	5	3.0
Roots and tuber	100	80	1.3	19	–
Green leafy vegetables	100	45	3.6	–	0.4
Other vegetables	100	30	1.7	–	0.2
Fruits	100	40	–	10	–
Sugar	5	20	–	5	–
Fats and oils	5	45	–	–	5

Table 4: Balanced diet for adults: Sedentary/moderate/heavy activity (number of portion).

Food group	Portion g	Type of work					
		Sedentary		Moderate		Heavy	
Cereals and millets	30	14	10	16	12	23	16
Pulses	30	2	2	3	2.5	3	3
Milk	100 mL	3	3	3	3	3	3
Roots and tubers	100	2	1	2	1	2	2
Other vegetables	100	1	1	1	1	1	1
Fruits	100	1	1	1	1	1	1
Sugar	5	5	4	8	5	11	9
Fats and oils (visible)	5	4	4	7	6	11	8

For non- vegetarians substitute one pulse portion with one portion of egg/meat/chicken/fish.
For infants introduce egg/meat/chicken/fish around 9 months.
Specific recommendations as compared to a sedentary women.

Children	
1–6 Years	½ to ¾ the amount of cereals, pulses and vegetables and extra cup of milk
7–12 years	Extra cup of milk
Adolescent girls	Extra cup of milk
Adolescent boys	Diet of sedentary man with extra cup of milk

Table 5: Balanced diet for infants, children and adolescents (number of portions).

Food groups	Portion g	Infants 6–12 months	\multicolumn{6}{c}{Years}

Food groups	Portion g	Infants 6–12 months	1–3	4–6	7–9	10–12 Girls	10–12 Boys	13–18 Girls	13–18 Boys
Cereals and millets	30	1.5	4	7	9	9	11	10	14
Pulses	30	0.5	1	1.5	2	2	2	2	2
Milk (mL)	100	5	5	5	5	5	5	5	5
Roots and tubers	100	0.5	0.5	1	1	1	1	1	1
Green leafy vegetables	100	0.25	0.5	0.5	1	1	1	1	1
Other vegetables	100	0.25	0.5	0.5	1	1	1	1	1
Fruits	100	1	1	1	1	1	1	1	1
Sugar	5	5	5	6	6	6	7	6	7
Fats/oils	5	2	4	5	5	5	5	5	5

There is no fat exchange as the calorie value of the recipes include fat that is used. If additional fat or sugar is used, calorie value can be calculated by multiplying with 9 or 4 per gram respectively.

All the food portion in the given list provide approximately the same amount of kilocalories. Portion sizes are strictly defined so that every item on a given list provides roughly the same amount of energy. Any food on a list can be exchanged for any other food on that same list without affecting a plan's balance or total calories.

Recipes from exchange lists are selected from all groups and energy and protein value are calculated in accordance with the RDA. If specific number of exchange lists are chosen from each group and energy and protein RDA are met, most of the time all the other nutrients are also met **(Table 6)**.

Table 6: Exchange list capacity of one standard calorie is 150 mL.	
Idli (big)	1
Idli (medium)	1 ⅓
Dosa (small)	1
Dosa (big)	½
Phulka	2
Chapati	1
Puri	1 ½
Rava idli	1
Veg sandwich	¾
Bread toast (medium)	1 ½
Bread pakoda	3
Plain rice	¾ kg
Upma	½ kg
Veg. noodles	1 kg
Coconut rice	½ kg
Pongal	½ kg
Boiled wheat rava	1 kg
Sweet pongal	2 Tb Sp
Raniyaram	1 ¼ Tb Sp
Vermicelli payasam	2 Tb Sp
Kesari	1 ½ Tb Sp
Rice flakes upma	½ kg
Naan	2/3
Cheese sandwich	1/3
Ragi puttu	¾ kg
Ragi adai	¾
Pulao	½ kg
Bise bela bath	½ kg
Tamarind rice	½ kg
Curd rice	½ kg
Idiappam	1

Contd...

Contd...

Pulse exchange—3–5 g protein	
Sambar	½ kg
Rasam	2 ½ kg
Thick dal	½ kg
Thin dal	1 kg
Channa masala	½ kg
Dry peas sundal	¾ kg
Roasted bengal gram chutney (with negligible amount of fat)	½ kg
Aai	1
Vada	1
Keerai vada	¾
Bajji	2
Bonda	1
Meat Exchange – 5 g of protein	
Egg omelette	1
Scrambled egg	One egg
Fish kolambu	2/3 kg
Fish fry	1 small piece
Boiled egg with gravy	1/3 to ½ serving
Meat curry	1 serving
Egg custard	½ kg
Milk exchange—4.5 g protein	
Milk	150 mL—1 tea cup
Curd	150 mL—1 full katori
Cheese	1 ⅓ cube 30 g
Paneer	40 g
Butter milk	1 glass – (350 mL)
Banana milk shake	¼ glass
Banna milk shake	1/3 glass
Milk kheer	½ kg
Carrot kheer	¾ kg

Healthy Diet

KEY FACTS

- A healthy diet helps to protect against malnutrition in all its forms, as well as non-communicable diseases (NCDs), including diabetes, heart disease, stroke and cancer.
- Unhealthy diet and lack of physical activity are leading global risks to health.
- Healthy dietary practices start early in life—breastfeeding fosters healthy growth and improves cognitive development, and may have longer-term health benefits, like reducing the risk of becoming overweight or obese and developing NCDs later in life.
- Energy intake (calories) should be in balance with energy expenditure. Evidence indicates that total fat should not exceed 30% of total energy intake to avoid unhealthy weight gain, with a shift in fat consumption away from saturated fats to unsaturated fats, and towards the elimination of industrial trans fats.
- Limiting intake of free sugars to less than 10% of total energy intake is part of a healthy diet. A further reduction to less than 5% of total energy intake is suggested for additional health benefits.
- Keeping salt intake to less than 5 g per day helps prevent hypertension and reduces the risk of heart disease and stroke in the adult population.
- WHO Member States have agreed to reduce the global population's intake of salt by 30% and halt the rise in diabetes and obesity in adults and adolescents as well as in childhood overweight by 2025.

OVERVIEW

Consuming a healthy diet throughout the life course helps to prevent malnutrition in all its forms as well as a range of non-communicable diseases and conditions. But the increased production of processed food, rapid urbanization and changing lifestyles have led to a shift in dietary patterns. People are now consuming more foods high in energy, fats, free sugars or salt/sodium, and many do not eat enough fruit, vegetables and dietary fiber such as whole grains.

The exact make-up of a diversified, balanced and healthy diet will vary depending on individual needs (e.g. age, gender, lifestyle, degree of physical activity), cultural context, locally available foods and dietary customs. But basic principles of what constitute a healthy diet remain the same.

For Adults

A healthy diet contains:
- Fruits, vegetables, legumes (e.g. lentils, beans), nuts and whole grains (e.g. unprocessed maize, millet, oats, wheat, brown rice).
- At least 400 g (5 portions) of fruits and vegetables a day. Potatoes, sweet potatoes, cassava and other starchy roots are not classified as fruits or vegetables.
- Less than 10% of total energy intake from free sugars which is equivalent to 50 g (or around 12 level teaspoons) for a person of healthy body weight consuming approximately 2000 calories per day, but ideally less than 5% of total energy intake for additional health benefits. Most free sugars are added to foods or drinks by the manufacturer, cook or consumer, and can also be found in sugars naturally present in honey, syrups, fruit juices and fruit juice concentrates.
- Less than 30% of total energy intake from fats. Unsaturated fats (e.g. those found in fish, avocado, nuts, sunflower, canola and olive oils) are preferable to saturated fats (e.g. found in fatty meat, butter, palm and coconut oil, cream, cheese, ghee and lard). Industrial trans fats (found in processed food, fast food, snack food, fried food, frozen pizza, pies, cookies, margarines and spreads) are not part of a healthy diet.
- Less than 5 g of salt (equivalent to approximately 1 teaspoon) per day and use iodized salt.

For Infants and Young Children

In the first 2 years of a child's life, optimal nutrition fosters healthy growth and improves cognitive development. It also reduces the risk of becoming overweight or obese and developing non-communicable diseases (NCDs) later in life.

Advice on a healthy diet for infants and children is similar to that for adults, but the following elements are also important:
- Infants should be breastfed exclusively during the first 6 months of life.
- Infants should be breastfed continuously until 2 years of age and beyond.
- From 6 months of age, breast milk should be complemented with a variety of adequate, safe and nutrient dense complementary foods. Salt and sugars should not be added to complementary foods.

Practical Advice on Maintaining a Healthy Diet

Fruits and Vegetables

Eating at least 400 g, or 5 portions, of fruits and vegetables per day reduces the risk of NCDs, and helps ensure an adequate daily intake of dietary fiber.

In order to improve fruit and vegetable consumption you can:
- Always include vegetables in your meals
- Eat fresh fruits and raw vegetables as snacks
- Eat fresh fruits and vegetables in season.
- Eat a variety of choices of fruits and vegetables.

Fats

Reducing the amount of total fat intake to less than 30% of total energy intake helps prevent unhealthy weight gain in the adult population.

Also, the risk of developing NCDs is lowered by reducing saturated fats to less than 10% of total energy intake, and trans fats to less than 1% of total energy intake, and replacing both with unsaturated fats.

Fat intake can be reduced by:
- Changing how you cook – remove the fatty part of meat; use vegetable oil (not animal oil); and boil, steam or bake rather than fry;
- Avoiding processed foods containing trans fats; and
- Limiting the consumption of foods containing high amounts of saturated fats (e.g. cheese, ice cream, fatty meat).

Salt, Sodium and Potassium

Most people consume too much sodium through salt (corresponding to an average of 9–12 g of salt per day) and not enough potassium. High salt consumption and insufficient potassium intake (less than 3.5 g) contribute to high blood pressure, which in turn increases the risk of heart disease and stroke.

1.7 million deaths could be prevented each year if people's salt consumption reduced to the recommended level of less than 5 g per day.

People are often unaware of the amount of salt they consume. In many countries, most salt comes from processed foods (e.g. ready meals; processed meats like bacon, ham and salami; cheese and salty snacks) or from food consumed frequently in large amounts (e.g. bread). Salt is also added to food during cooking (e.g. bouillon, stock cubes, soy sauce and fish sauce) or at the table (e.g. table salt).

You can reduce salt consumption by:
- Not adding salt, soy sauce or fish sauce during the preparation of food
- Not having salt on the table
- Limiting the consumption of salty snacks
- Choosing products with lower sodium content.

Some food manufacturers are reformulating recipes to reduce the salt content of their products, and it is helpful to check food labels to see how much sodium is in a product before purchasing or consuming it.

Potassium, which can mitigate the negative effects of elevated sodium consumption on blood pressure, can be increased with consumption of fresh fruits and vegetables.

Sugars

The intake of free sugars should be reduced throughout the lifecourse. Evidence indicates that in both adults and children, the intake of free sugars should be reduced to less than 10% of total energy intake, and that a reduction to less than 5% of total energy intake provides additional health benefits. Free sugars are all sugars added to foods or drinks by the manufacturer, cook or consumer, as well as sugars naturally present in honey, syrups, fruit juices and fruit juice concentrates.

Consuming free sugars increases the risk of dental caries (tooth decay). Excess calories from foods and drinks high in free sugars also contribute to unhealthy weight gain, which can lead to overweight and obesity.

Sugars intake can be reduced by:
- Limiting the consumption of foods and drinks containing high amounts of sugars (e.g. sugar-sweetened beverages, sugary snacks and candies); and
- Eating fresh fruits and raw vegetables as snacks instead of sugary snacks.

3 Minor Ailments and Home Remedies

INTRODUCTION

Minor ailments are generally defined as conditions that will resolve on their own and can be reasonably self-diagnosed. Minor ailments include common conditions such as headaches, back pain, insect bites, diaper rash, heartburn or indigestion, nasal congestion, etc. While most individuals self-manage minor ailments with over-the-counter medications, it is estimated that general practitioners spend approximately 18 percent or more of their time treating clients with these types of condition.

HOUSEHOLD CURES

Throughout the world, household or home remedies are used; often, traditional ways of healing have been passed down from generations to generations. Some are useful; some are less useful while others can be risky or harmful. Therefore, household or home remedies must be used with caution. For many sicknesses, time-tested household remedies work as well as modern medicines or even better; in some cases, they are often cheaper and safer. Home remedies help some diseases, while others are better treated with modern medicines. This is true for most serious infections like pneumonia, typhoid, tetanus, tuberculosis, appendicitis, sexually transmitted diseases and so on. For others like diabetes, hypertension, heart and kidney diseases, must see a medical practitioner. For these diseases, do not waste time or risk life trying home remedies.

There is no medicine that does not have some risk in its use. Therefore, it is safer to treat very serious ailments with modern medicines following advice of a medical doctor or a pharmacist.

Diarrhea and Vomiting–Water

If a child or baby has a sudden bout of watery diarrhea and/or vomiting, take them off solids and milk and offer plenty of clear fluids or electrolyte fluid. If baby is breastfed, continue breastfeeding.

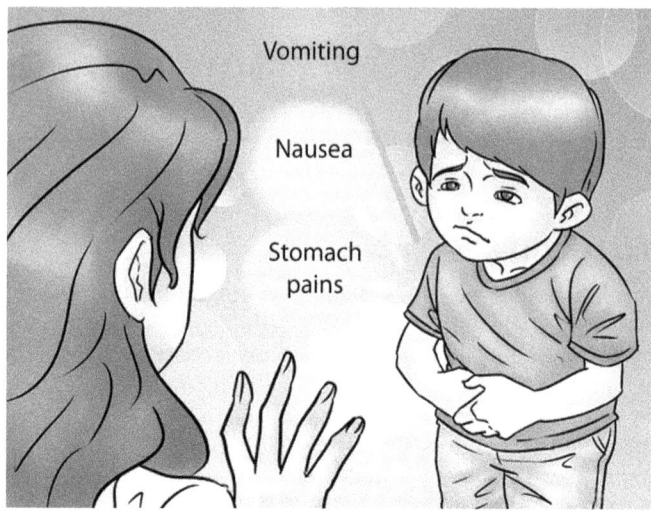

Fig. 1: Signs and symptoms of diarrhea.

Advice a diet of rice water, coconut water, etc.

Teach mother to use diapers for the children to prevent further spread of the disease.

If the symptoms are severe, or the child continues to vomit for more than 12-24 hours, refer to primary health center (PHC).

The same principles apply to adults. Offer frequent clear fluids or electrolyte fluid.

Stomach Ulcers and Acid Indigestion

Drink diluted milk several times a day especially at the end of each meal.

Avoid the following: Alcoholic drinks, coffee, cigarettes, pepper and other spices, carbonated drinks (e.g. cola drinks and soda water).

Avoid anger, tension and nervousness which make ulcers worse.

Constipation

- Drink plenty of water.
- Eat fruits, vegetables and foods with natural fiber.
- In the elderly, there is need to do some exercise (e.g. walking) in order to have regular bowel movement.
- If there has been no bowel movement for three or more days even after the above precautions, refer to PHC.

Chapter 3 Minor Ailments and Home Remedies

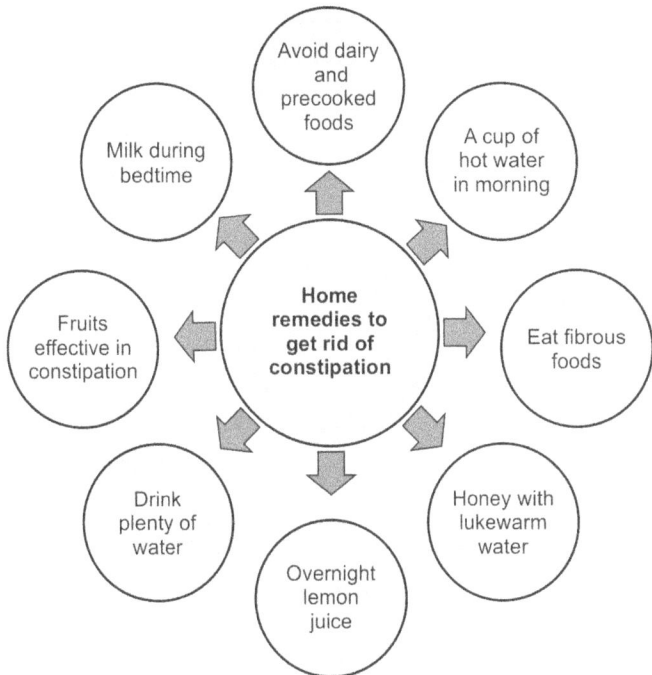

Fig. 2: Home remedies of constipation.

Control of Simple Vomiting
- Eat nothing while vomiting is severe.
- Sip a ginger ale or rehydration drink.

Fever

To treat, manage and control a fever, the following procedure should be taken:

The client should be uncovered and fanned. It is dangerous to cover a client with fever with thick clothes. Small children should be left naked until the fever goes down. The child may also be bathed in cold water if the fever is high. For babies and small children, the water should be boiled and cooled. Find and treat the cause of the fever.

A child will develop a hot temperature because of an infection. Dress child in cool clothes. Leave the child's head uncovered. Open doors and windows till the child feels better and the temperature is lowered. If child does not improve after giving sponging or appears particularly ill, refer to PHC.

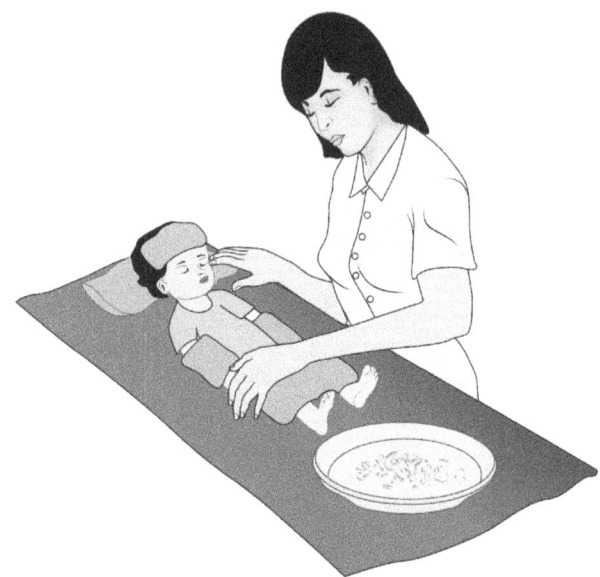

Fig. 3: Cold compress at home.

Headaches

Most headaches are due to simple causes ranging from tension and eye strain to migraine, take rest and relaxation is usually all that is needed. Or take a lime, cut it in half and rub on forehead.

Coughs

Cough medicines do not cure coughs! (coughs with runny noses are usually caused by viruses for which there is no cure.) Coughs may be soothed by cough medicines bought at the chemist or by a drink made from honey and freshly squeezed lemon juice in hot water which is cheaper. Cough sweets (not for children) may also soothe tickly coughs until they run their course. If cough persists for more than seven days and bring up colored phlegm, or were wheezing, need to see physician.

Children with coughs who may have a runny nose, are a little off color, not eating or vomiting with the strength of coughing or have a temperature but are otherwise all right, should be treated as above. In addition, they should also have their temperature controlled and be given small amounts of fluids, such as salt-sugar solution (ORT) regularly.

Chapter 3 Minor Ailments and Home Remedies **59**

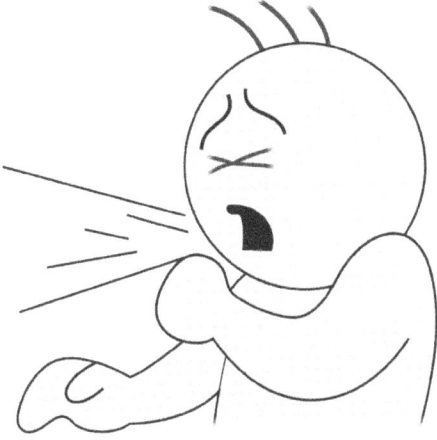

Fig. 4: Respiratory infection.

Burns

Remove the person from the danger. Cool the burnt area by holding it under cold, running water or immerse the area in cold water until the pain subsides. This should take at least 10 to 15 minutes. If the skin is unbroken but blistered, apply a cold water soak dressing and seek medical attention. This also applies if the skin is unbroken. (Never Break Blisters Caused By A Burn).

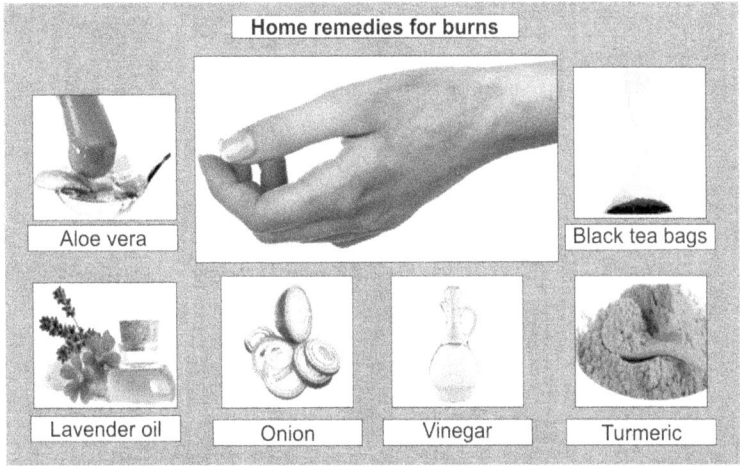

Fig. 5: Home remedies for burn.

Colds

Drink plenty of fluid and go to bed (water based drinks are best).

Sprains

As well as pain, there will probably be bruising and swelling. Apply a cold compress, containing ice if possible, for 15 to 30 minutes to reduce the swelling. Bandage firmly, and give the sprain plenty of rest until the discomfort has subsided. Further strain will lead to added swelling and a longer recovery period.

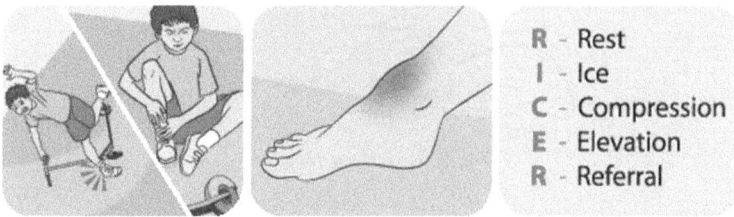

Fig. 6: Sprain manangement.

Nose Bleeds

Sit the client down with their head tilted forward over a bowl. While the Client breathes through their mouth, pinch their nose just below the bone for about 10 minutes. The bleeding should stop.

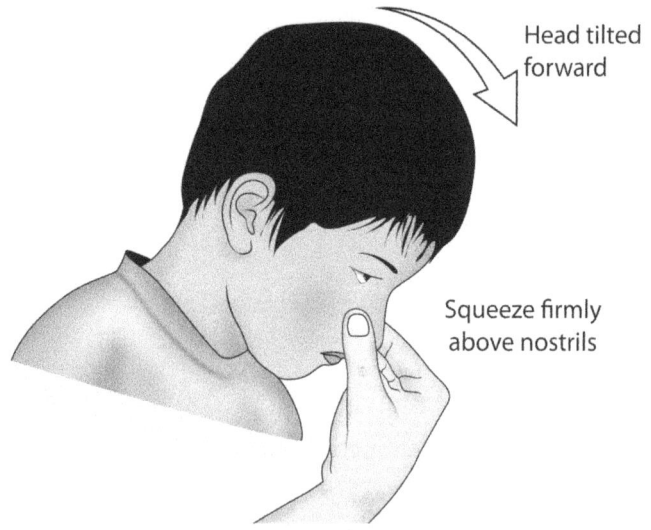

Fig. 7: Care of nose bleeding.

Chapter 3 Minor Ailments and Home Remedies 61

Minor Cuts and Grazes

If the wound is dirty, rinse it under cold running water and clean around it with soap and water, wiping away from the wound. To stop bleeding, apply a clean dressing firmly to the wound for about five minutes. Cover with a clean dry dressing and Never put cotton wool directly into an open wound.

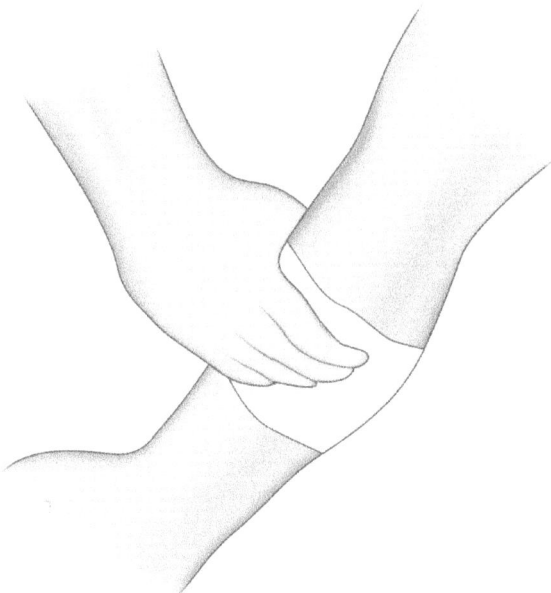

Fig. 8: Minor cut manangement.

Insect Bites and Stings

Bees leave their stings in, so first priority is to carefully remove the sting. Bee stings should be scraped away rather than 'plucked' to avoid squeezing the contents of the venom sac into the wound.

Head Lice

Contrary to popular belief, head lice prefer clean hair and are, therefore, not a sign of poor personal hygiene. There are a number of options available to treat head lice. Ask doctor for details.

Back Pain

For the first few days rest back by lying on a firm mattress placed either on the floor or on wooden boards between the mattress and the base of bed. Apply gentle heat, e.g. from a hot water bottle or heat lamp will often help. As the pain begins to ease, start gentle exercises as soon as possible even if can only move back a few inches in each direction. Avoid straining back while exercising and take great care when lifting even if the pain has completely settled. When sitting, an upright chair with the support for the small of the back puts much less strain on spine.

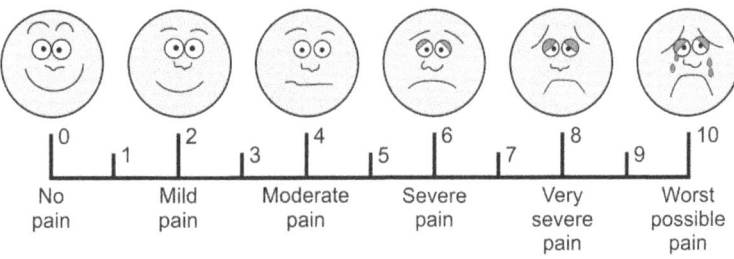

Fig. 9: Pain scale.

Animal Bite

Wash the wound with soap and water for animal bites other than dog bite. Seek medical aid. Refer to primary health centre.

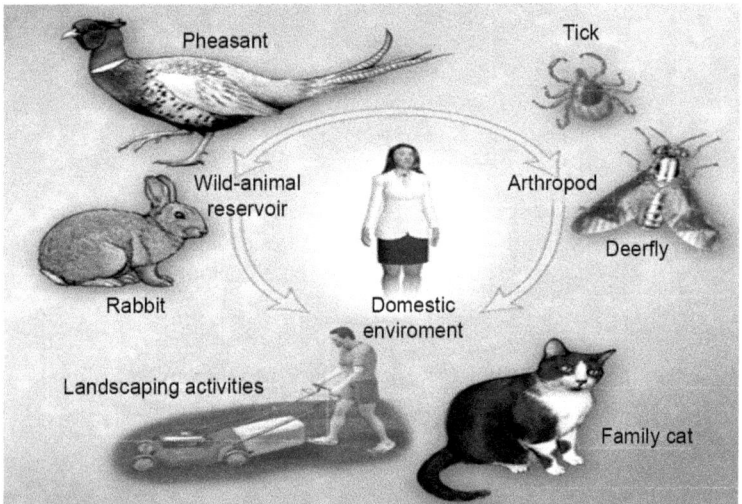

Fig. 10: Common animal bites.

Conjunctivitis

This is an infection that makes the eyes red, sore and often with watery discharge (like tears). It often settles without treatment if bath the eyes with boiled water and wipe away the 'matter' with clean cotton wool. If it does not settle, consult a doctor. It is often very infectious, so Clients should never share towels and should wash their hands with soap and water immediately after touching their eyes.

4 Individual, Family, Community and Wellness Diagnoses

INTRODUCTION
Creating nursing diagnoses requires the application of detailed assessment skills, critical thinking, and decision making. The formulation of nursing diagnoses is related to competency in diagnostic reasoning which students begin in their first year.

DEFINITIONS
A diagnosis is a statement that synthesizes (brings together) assessment data. It is a label that describes a situation (or state) and implies an etiology (reason) and gives evidence to support the inference.

- Caregiver role strain related to caring for family member with diabetes mellitus
  - Assess the caregiver stress level
  - Explain the progressive nature of the diseases
  - Instruct the caregiver to encourage client to participate in social and self-care activity
  - Facilitate the family meeting to help the primary caregiver seek assistance from other family members
  - Help the caregiver contact informal sources of support, such as religious groups, extended family, and community volunteers for support and relief
- Ineffective community coping related to increased level of teen pregnancy
  - Assess the teenager's knowledge about sex and sexuality to determine their education needs.
  - Work with schools to develop pregnancy prevention programs
  - Work closely with individual pregnant adolescents to assess their needs and provide care
  - Plan for an outreach program to raise community members awareness of the need to approach teen pregnancy as a community problem
  - Conduct mass health education programs

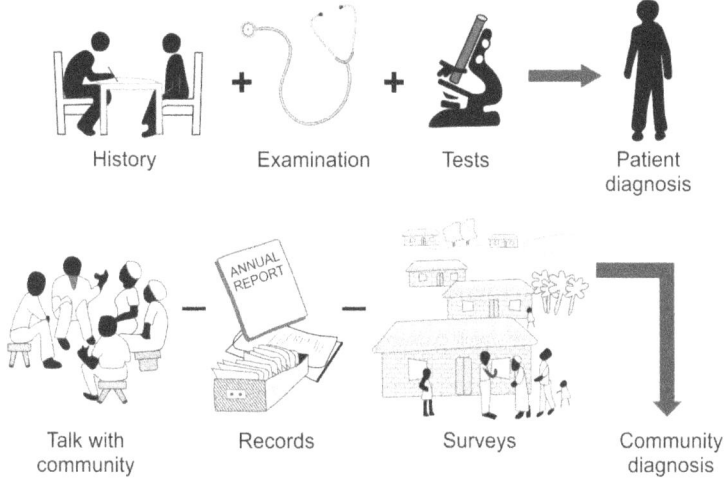

Fig. 1: Steps of nursing care in community.

- Readiness for enhanced community coping related to immunization
  - Assess the potential problems associated with inadequate immunization
  - Identify new members of the community such as immigrants, to help reach parents who need information on immunization
  - Provide extensive health education on communicable diseases and its importance of immunization
  - Contacts the parents of children who are not immunized person
  - Provide immunization information in parents first language to overcome a lack of understanding caused by language barriers.
- Anticipatory grieving related to the need for hospice care
  - Assess the client and his family members psycho-social status
  - Clarify their all queries
  - Check vital signs periodically and note the complicated sign
  - Encourage the client to make simple decisions related to his care
  - Explain the client and family members about pain control, comfort measures, diet etc.
  - Support the client spiritual coping behavior.
- Delayed growth and development related to environmental and stimulation deficiencies
  - Assess the psycho-social status
  - Help teachers, staff members, and administrators identify students who may at high risk

- Educate teachers about each students condition and about the adaptation needed in the classroom
- Encourage parents, teachers and staff members to identify socially skilled children and to encourage the children to participate in group activities
- Work with parents and teachers to initiate activities among children that encourage interaction in small groups.
- Risk for infection related to home infusion therapy
  - Assess the health status of the client
  - Provide care in systematic way
  - Ensure the patient and caregiver understand the purpose of treatment and enlist the participation throughout the therapy
  - Provide emotional support
  - Provide all necessary supplies
  - Emphasize the importance of safety precaution
  - Explain about the management of complication
- Risk for infection related to increase incidence of tuberculosis
  - Assess for a history of exposure to tuberculosis. Or physical evidence of exposure
  - Refer the high risk individual to the nearby PHC
  - Emphasize the need to take drugs exactly as prescribed
  - Teach the client about the potential effects of medication to encourage the client to recognize and report adverse effect promptly
  - Teach about the safety precautions to be followed.
- Deficient knowledge related to familiarity with managed care
  - Assess the educational status of the client
  - Provide a simple explanation of managed care
  - Explain about the positive and negatives outcome of the illness
  - Encourage clients to ask questions and clarify it
  - Reassess the client knowledge.
- High risk for infection related to poor environmental sanitation
  - Assess the environmental surrounding
  - Teach about the cleanliness of the community
  - Educate them to avoid open drainage system
  - Advice the people to keep the utensils and vessels closed
  - Encourage to drink boiled water
- Infective community therapeutic regimen management related to drug and alcohol abuse among teenagers
  - Assess the demographics of the population
  - Assess the prevalence of the health problems

Chapter 4 Individual, Family, Community and Wellness... 67

- Work with Accredited Social Health Activist (ASHA), Anganwadi teachers and leaders to make awareness of the drug abuse
- Encourage the youth association to emphasize the importance of alcohol and its impact among alcoholics
- Counsel and do mass health education in the community.
- Imbalanced nutrition less than body requirement related to lack of resources or knowledge
  - Assess the nutritional status of the client
  - Draw a menu plan
  - Advice the client to have high protein and calorie rich diet
  - Check the weight of the client
  - Provide small and frequent diets.
- Pain management
  - Assess the pain characteristic of pain
  - Advice to have healthy diet
  - Avoid heavy weight lifting
  - Psychological support
  - Hot and cold application.
- Sleep pattern disturbance
  - Assess the sleep pattern of the client
  - Advice to avoid day time sleep.
  - Provide calm and quite environment
  - Provide warm milk before sleep
  - Advice to void before go to bed.
- Activity intolerance
  - Assess the activity of the client
  - Advice the family members to assist the client
  - Encourage to do mild activities
  - Client should take adequate rest
  - Keep the need things near him/her.
- Risk for suicidal tendency related to poor family support
  - Assess the psychological status of the client
  - Do mental status examination
  - Provide psychological support
  - Educate the family to support the client
  - Refer to hospital.
- Ineffective airway clearance related to increased secretion
  - Assess the general condition
  - Check the respiratory rate
  - Comfortable position with devices
  - Advice to avoid exposure to cold
  - Provide thulsi extract.

- Hyperthermia related to infection
  - Assess the general condition
  - Check the temperature
  - Tepid sponge for adults/cold compress for child
  - Advice to consume boiled water
  - Administer medication as per standing order.

5

Checklist

Checklist for Conducting Normal Delivery (Second Stage of Labor), Essential Newborn Care (ENBC) and Active Management of Third Stage of Labor (AMTSL)

S. No.	Task	Cases				
		1	2	3	4	5

1.	*Getting ready*
	• Keep the equipment, supplies and drugs necessary for conducting a delivery ready:
	For the provider
	• Plastic apron, mask, shoe covers, goggles-1 each
	• High level disinfection (HLD)/sterile gloves (no. 6½/7/7½)-2 pairs according to size of provider's hand
	• Functional light source
	For the mother and the baby
	• Delivery table with mattress, pillow and disposable/linen sheet, Galli's pot and foot stool
	• BP instrument and stethoscope—1 each and functional
	• Fetoscope—1
	• Thermometer—1
	• Plastic sheet—1
	• Pre-warmed towels for the baby—2
	• Clock with second's hand on the wall—1
	• Woman's record and partograph
	• Measuring tape—1
	• Adhesive tape—1
	• Delivery tray with lid containing:
	  – Sponge holding forceps—1
	  – Artery forceps-2 and scissors—1
	  – Urinary catheter (plain)—1
	  – Cord ligatures-3 or cord clamp—1
	  – De Lees mucus extractor—1					

Contd...

Contd...

- Stainless steel kidney tray 10 inches or SS bowl 10 inches diameter—1
- Pads for mother—4
- Sterile disposable needle and syringe 2 mL—1
- Oxytocin injection-10 IU loaded in the sterile syringe/misoprostol tablets 600 mcg (out of the tray)
- Injection vit. K loaded in a sterile syringe for the baby
• IV stand, IV set, normal saline/ringers lactate—1 each

Infection prevention equipment and supplies
- Swabs/pieces of gauze—at least 6–10
- Small bowl for cotton swabs and antiseptic lotion
- Antiseptic solution (Povidone Iodine) freshly poured on the swabs
- Leak proof container to dispose soiled linen—1
- Puncture proof container to discard needle and syringe—1/needle and hub cutter—1
- Color coded plastic containers with biodegradable plastic liners to dispose of the placenta, contaminated and biomedical waste—1 each as per government guidelines
- Plastic container with 0.5% chlorine solution for decontamination—1

Baby resuscitation equipment and tray ready for use if required
Radiant warmer switched on half an hour prior to delivery

Sterile episiotomy tray with its contents should be available in the labor room for use if indicated

Medicine and emergency drug trays to be available in the labor room and postpartum intrauterine contraceptive device (PPIUCD) tray in the labor room of facilities with PPIUCD trained providers

• Allows the woman to adopt the position of her choice
• Maintains privacy
• Tells the woman and her support person what is going to be done and encourages them to ask questions
• Listens to what the woman and her support person have to say
• Provides emotional support and reassurance

Contd...

Contd...

2.	*Conduction of delivery*:
	• Removes all the jewelry, watch and puts on a clean plastic apron, mask, goggles and shoes/shoe covers
	• Places one clean plastic sheet from the delivery kit under the woman's buttocks
	• Washes hands thoroughly with soap and water, air dries them
	• Wears sterile/HLD gloves on both the hands and cleans the perineal area from above downward with cotton swabs dipped in antiseptic lotion
	
	Delivery of the head once crowning occurs:
	• Keeps one hand gently on the head under the sub-pubic angle as it advances with the contractions to maintain flexion
	• Supports the perineum with the other hand and covers the anus with a pad held in position by the hand
	• Tells the mother to take deep breaths and to bear down only during a contraction
	• Once the head is out, uses gauze to gently wipe the mucus off the baby's face
	• Feels gently around the baby's neck for the presence of the umbilical cord, checks:
	   – If the cord is present and is loose around the neck, delivers the baby through the loop of the cord, or slips the cord over the baby's head
	   – If the cord is tight around the neck, places two artery clamps on the cord and cuts between the clamps, and then unwinds it from around the neck
	
	Delivery of the shoulders and the rest of the body:
	• Waits for spontaneous rotation of the head and shoulders and delivery of the shoulders. This usually happens within 1–2 minutes
	• Applies gentle pressure downwards on the shoulder under the sub-pubic arch to deliver the top (anterior) shoulder
	• Then lifts the baby up, towards the mother's abdomen, to deliver the lower (posterior) shoulder
	• The rest of the baby's body follows smoothly by lateral flexion				

Contd...

Contd...

Essential newborn care (ENBC) and initiation of Active management of third stage of labor (AMTSL):			
• Notes the sex and time of birth • Places the baby on the mother's abdomen in a prone position with face to one side • Looks for breathing or crying of the baby. If the baby is breathing or crying, proceeds immediately to dry the baby with a pre-warmed towel or piece of clean cloth. (Does not wipe off the white greasy substance–vernix, covering the baby's body) • After drying, discards the wet towel or cloth after wiping the mother's abdomen also • Wraps the baby loosely in another clean, dry and warm towel. If the baby remains wet, it leads to heat loss • *Initiates AMTSL*: Palpates the mother's abdomen to feel for fetal parts to exclude the presence of another baby to initiate the active management of third stage of labor • *Uterotonic drug*: Gives 10 units Oxytocin IM in the anterolateral aspect of the woman's thigh if she is at the health facility (preferred) or gives misoprostol tablets (600 mcg that is 3 tablets of 200 mcg each or a single tablet of 600 mcg) if it is a home delivery and oxytocin is not available • Completes drying and wrapping of the crying baby and giving injection Oxytocin within the first minute after birth of the baby • *Continues ENBC*: Checks for cord pulsations • Clamps the cord with artery clamps at two places when cord pulsations stop. Puts one clamp on the cord at least 3 cm away from the baby's umbilicus and the other clamp 5 cm from the baby's umbilicus. • Cuts the cord between the artery clamps with a sterile scissors by placing a sterile gauze over the cord and scissors to prevent splashing of blood • Applies the disposable sterile plastic cord clamp tightly on the cord 2 cm away from the umbilicus just before the artery clamp (instrument) and removes the artery clamp on the side of the baby's abdomen; gently places and directs the other clamped cord end towards the contaminated waste bin under the labor table to avoid spillage			

Contd...

Contd...

	• In the absence of sterile disposable cord clamp, ties, clean thread ties tightly around the cord at approximately 2–3 cm and 5 cm from the baby's abdomen and cuts between the ties with a sterile, clean blade. If there is oozing, places a second tie between the baby's skin and the first tie • Gives injection vitamin K intramuscular to the baby • Places the baby between the mother's breasts for warmth and skin to skin care. Tells the mother or the attendant to hold the baby in place to prevent falling • Puts the identification tag on the baby. Covers the baby's head with a cloth. Covers the mother and the baby with a warm cloth.				

3.	Continues active management of third stage of labor (AMTSL):
	• *Controlled cord traction (CCT)*: (attempts only when the uterus is contracted)
	  – Assures the woman that delivering the placenta will not hurt, because it is much smaller and softer than the baby
	  – Clamps the maternal end of the umbilical cord close to the perenium with an artery clamp
	  – Holds the clamped end with one hand and places the other hand just above the symphysis pubis, for counter traction on the uterus to prevent inversion
	  – Holds the cord with the help of the clamp and waits for a contraction
	  – Only during contractions, gently pulls the cord downwards and then downwards and forwards to deliver the placenta
	  – With the other hand, pushes the uterus upwards by applying counter traction. (If the placenta does not descend within 30–40 seconds of CCT, does not continue to pull on the cord. Waits for about 5 more minutes for the uterus to contract strongly, then repeats CCT with counter traction)
	  – As the placenta appears at the vaginal introitus, holds it with both hands and twists it clockwise to deliver it complete and prevents tearing of the membranes				

Contd...

Contd...

	– Gently keeps twisting the placenta with membranes so that they get twisted in to a rope and are expelled and slip out of the introitus intact and complete – Places the placenta in a tray *Uterine massage*: • Places the cupped palm on the uterine fundus and feels for the state of contraction • If the uterus is soft and not-contracted, massages the uterine fundus in a circular motion with the cupped palm until the uterus is well contracted. A well contracted uterus feels like a cricket ball or the forehead • When the uterus is well contracted, places her fingers behind the fundus and pushes down in one swift action to expel clots • Estimates and records the amount of blood loss approximately • Encourages the attendant to help the woman to breastfeed *Examination of the lower vagina and perineum*. • Ensures that adequate light is falling on the perenium • With gloved hands, gently separates the labia and inspects the perineum and vagina for bleeding, laceration/tears • If lacerations/tears are present, manages them as per the protocols [will be dealt with in detail during postpartum hemorrhage [PPH] • Cleans the vulva and perineum gently with warm water or an antiseptic solution and dries with a clean soft cloth • Places a pad or clean, sun-dried cloth on the woman's perineum • Removes soiled linen to make the woman comfortable and shifts her up to lie comfortably on the delivery table *Examination of the placenta, membranes and the umbilical cord*: • Maternal surface of the placenta: – Holds the placenta in the palms of the hands, keeping the palms flat. Makes sure the maternal surface is facing up – Checks if all the lobules are present and fit together				

Contd...

Contd...

- After the maternal side has been rinsed carefully with water, it should shine because of the decidual covering
- If any of the lobes is missing or the lobules do not fit together, suspects that some placental fragments may have been left behind in the uterus
- *Fetal surface*:
  - Holds the umbilical cord in one hand and lets the placenta and membranes hang down like an inverted umbrella
  - Looks for holes which may indicate that a part of the lobe has been left behind in the uterus
  - Looks for the point of insertion of the cord, the point where it is inserted into the membranes and from where it travels to the placenta
- *Membranes*:
  - Puts one hand inside the membranes to open them and see for any holes or irregular edges other than the one from where the membranes ruptured and the baby came out
  - Places the membranes together and makes sure that they are complete
- *Umbilical cord*:
  - Inspects the umbilical cord for two arteries and one vein. If only one artery is found, looks for congenital malformations in the baby
- *Decontamination and disposal of waste*:
  - Disposes the placenta in the yellow colored contaminated waste bin after removing the artery clamp
  - Places the instruments used in 0.5% chlorine solution for 10 minutes for decontamination
  - Decontaminates or disposes of the syringes and needles
  - Immerses both the gloved hands in 0.5% chlorine solution
    - Removes the gloves by turning them inside out
    - For disposing of the gloves, places them in a leak proof container or red plastic bin
    - If the surgical gloves are to be re-used, submerges them in 0.5% chlorine solution for 10 minutes to decontaminate them
- Washes hands thoroughly with soap and water and air dries
- Completes the records of the woman

Contd...

Contd...

Prepare for newborn resuscitation (NBR) if required:
Immediately after birth—
• If the baby is not crying or not breathing, irrespective if the meconium is present or not, quickly applies suction to the mouth and then the nose to clear the airways while the baby is on the mother's abdomen and quickly dries the baby with the warm towel
• Assesses the baby's breathing:
  – If the baby starts breathing well and the chest is rising regularly, between 30–60 times a minute, provides routine care
  – If the baby is still not breathing or is gasping, calls for help. Clamps the cord immediately, even before 1 minute and asks the co-provider to take the baby to the radiant warmer at the newborn care center (NBCC) in the labor room (LR) for further suction and resuscitation with bag and mask while she manages the third stage of labor
  – The steps of resuscitation (as described in the checklist for NBR) need to be carried out immediately
Immediate care of mother after delivery (within 2 hours of delivery near the labor room):
• Check the uterus and vaginal bleeding at least every 15 minutes for the first 2 hours, massaging as and when necessary to keep it hard. Make sure the uterus does not become soft (relaxed) after massage is discontinued. Ensure, the mother is comfortable and her vitals are normal.
• Ensure the baby is breathing normally. Check weight of the baby and gives injection Vitamin K intramuscular, 1 mg to > 1000 g baby and 0.5 g to the baby weighing < 1000 g in the anterolateral thigh to prevent hemorrhagic disease of the newborn.
• If both mother and baby are normal shift them together to the postpartum ward.				

Checklist for Newborn Resuscitation

S. No.	Task	Yes/No	Remarks
1.	Getting ready with: • Bag and masks (sizes '0' and '1') • Suction equipment • Radiant warmer or other heat source • Warm towels—2 • Clock with seconds hand • Oxygen source • Gloves • Shoulder roll • Cord tie • Scissor		
2.	Look for breathing, if not, suck mouth and nose at the mother's abdomen		
3.	Dry the baby, remove wet towel by cleaning the mothers' abdomen also and wrap baby in warm dry towel		
4.	Assess breathing, if not breathing or difficulty in breathing then-		
5.	Cut the cord immediately		
6.	Place the baby on a warm, firm flat surface (radiant warmer)		
7.	**P**osition the baby in slight neck extension using a shoulder roll **S**uction of mouth and nose **S**timulate the baby **R**eposition and reassess breathing		
8.	If not breathing provide bag and mask ventilation for 30 seconds, make sure that the chest rises.		
9.	Reassess the baby after 30 seconds of ventilation.		
10.	If still not breathing continue bag and mask ventilation, start oxygen and assess the heart rate.		
11.	If the baby is still not breathing, continue bag and mask ventilation and refer to higher center		
12.	At any point if baby starts breathing, provide observational care		

Checklist for Breastfeeding

S. No.	Steps	Observations
1.	Advice mother to sit or lie in comfortable position and help the mother to initiate breastfeeding	
2.	Advice for cleaning of nipples and breasts	
3.	Describe and demonstrate rooting reflex	
4.	Describe and ensure correct position • Baby's body is well supported • The head, neck and body of baby are kept in the same plane • Entire body of baby faces mother • Baby's abdomen touches mother's abdomen	
5.	Describe and ensure good attachment • Baby's mouth is wide abdomen • Lower lip is turned out • Chin is touching mother's breast • Larger area of areola is visible above than below	
6.	Describe and ensure effective suckling—slow deep sucks with pauses	
7.	Advice burping after breastfeeding	
8.	Inform the mother regarding frequency of feeding (at least 8 times in 24 hours including night feeds) and importance of emptying the breasts and hind milk	
9.	Inspect breasts for sore nipples, cuts and engorgement, actracted or inverted	
10.	Counsel on advantages of colostrum feeding and reinforce exclusive breastfeeding	
11.	Counsel regarding correct diet, adequate rest and stress free environment	

Checklist on Family Planning Counseling

Step/task (Some of the following steps/tasks should be performed simultaneously)	Cases				
Preparation for counseling					
1. Ensures room is well lit and there is availability of chairs and table					
2. Prepares equipment and supplies					
3. Ensures availability of writing materials (e.g. client file, daily activity register, follow-up cards)					
4. Ensures privacy					
General counseling skills					
1. Greets the woman with respect and kindness. Introduces self					
2. Confirms woman's name, address and other required information					
3. Offers the woman a place to sit. Ensures her comfort					
4. Reassures the woman that the information in the counseling session is confidential					
5. Tells the woman what is going to be done and encourages questions. Responds to the woman's questions/concerns					
6. Gives a brief description of the family planning methods available					
7. Uses body language to show interest in and concern for the woman					
8. Asks questions appropriately and with respect. Elicits more than "yes" and "no" answers					
9. Uses language that the woman can understand					
10. Appropriately uses visual aids, such as posters, flipcharts, drawings, samples of methods and anatomic models					
11. Discusses the health benefits to mother and baby of waiting at least two years after the birth of her last baby before she tries to conceive again					

Contd...

Contd...

Specific family planning counseling				
1.	Ask the woman if she has a method in mind. Did she have any problems with that method or does she have any question or concern about that method?			
2.	Ask the woman does she want more children			
3.	Discuss with the woman the benefits of healthy timing and spacing of pregnancy			
4.	Ask the woman if her husband will contribute to using family planning such as using condoms			
5.	Ask the woman if she is currently breastfeeding			
6.	Is she EBF, amenorrheic and her infant <6 months (LAM)?			
7.	Ask the woman what the first day of her last menses was			
8.	Ask the woman if she has any history of medical problems (TB, seizures, irregular vaginal bleeding, liver disease, unusual vaginal discharge and pelvic pain, clotting disorder, breast or genital cancer)			
9.	Assess the woman's risk for STIs and HIV/AIDS, as appropriate			
10.	Briefly, provide general information about each contraceptive method that is appropriate for that woman based on her responses to questions 1–9: • How to use the method • Effectiveness • Common side effects • Need for protection against STIs including HIV/AIDS			
11.	Clarifie any misinformation the woman may have about family planning methods			
12.	Ask which method interests the woman. Helps the woman chose a method			
Method-Specific Counseling–once the woman has chosen a method				
1.	Perform a physical assessment that is appropriate for the method chosen, if indicated, refers the woman for evaluation. (BP for hormonal, pelvic for IUCD)			

Contd...

Contd...

2.	Ensure there are no conditions that contraindicate the use of the chosen method. • If necessary, helps the woman to find a more suitable method					
3.	Tell the woman about the family planning method she has chosen: • Type • How to take it, and what to do if she is late taking her method • How it works • Effectiveness • Advantages and non-contraceptive benefits • Disadvantages • Common side effects • Danger signs and where to go if she experiences any					
4.	Provide the method of choice if available or refer woman to the nearest health facility where it is available					
5.	Ask the woman to repeat the instructions about her chosen method of contraception: How to use the method of contraception Side effects When to return to the clinic					
6.	Educate the woman about prevention of STIs and HIV/AIDS. Provide her with condoms if she is at risk					
7.	Ask if the woman has any questions or concerns. Listen attentively, addresse her questions and concerns					
8.	Schedule the follow-up visit. Encourages the woman to return to the clinic at any time if necessary					
9.	Records the relevant information in the woman's chart					
10.	Thank the woman politely, say goodbye and encourage her to return to the clinic if she has any questions or concerns					
Follow-up counseling						
1.	Greets the woman with respect and kindness. Introduces self					

Contd...

Contd...

2.	Confirm the woman's name, address and other required information					
3.	Ask the woman the purpose of her visit					
4.	Review her record/chart					
5.	Check whether the woman is satisfied with her family planning method and is still using it. Ask if she has any questions, concerns, or problems with the method					
6.	Explore changes in the woman's health status or lifestyle that may mean she needs a different family planning method					
7.	Reassure the woman about side effects she is having and treat them if necessary					
8.	Ask the woman if she has any questions. Listen to her attentively and responds to her questions or concerns					
9.	Perform any necessary physical assessment					
10.	Provide the woman with her contraceptive method (e.g. the pill, DMPA, condoms, etc.)					
11.	Schedule return visit as necessary—tell her. Thanks her politely and say goodbye • Record info in her chart					

Chapter 5 Checklist **83**

Checklist for Gestational Age Estimation

Abdominal Examination, Correct Estimation of Gestational Age					
S. No.	Task	Cases				
		1	2	3	4	5
1.	*Note*:					
	• It is important that abdominal examination during pregnancy be done with an empty bladder. Ask the woman to empty her bladder. • Give the woman a clean bottle and ask her to collect a little urine in the bottle before emptying her bladder completely. The urine will be required later to test for sugar and proteins. • Maintain privacy and obtain the woman's verbal consent.					
2.	Help the woman lie comfortably on her back, supported by cushions or pillows, on the examination table. Ask her to loosen her clothes and uncover her abdomen.					
3.	Check the abdomen for any scars. If there is a scar, find out if it is from a cesarean section or any other uterine surgery.					
4.	Fundal height					
	a. Ask the woman to keep her legs straight. b. Measuring fundal height To estimate the gestational age through the fundal height, the abdomen is divided into parts by imaginary lines. The most important line is the one passing through the umbilicus. Then divide the lower abdomen (below the umbilicus) into three parts, with two equidistant lines between the symphysis pubis and the umbilicus. Similarly, divide the upper abdomen into three parts, again with two imaginary equidistant lines, between the umbilicus and the xiphisternum.					
	At 12th week: Just palpable above the symphysis pubis					
	At 16th week: At lower one-third of the distance between the symphysis pubis and umbilicus					
	At 20th week: At two-thirds of the distance between the symphysis pubis and umbilicus					

Contd...

Contd...

At 24th week: At the level of the umbilicus				
At 28th week: At lower one-third of the distance between the umbilicus and xiphisternum				
At 32nd week: At two-third of the distance between the umbilicus and xiphisternum				
At 36th week: At the level of the xiphisternum				
At 40th week: Sinks back to the level of the 32nd week, but the flanks are full, unlike that in the 32nd week.				
c. Measuring FH (in cm) using Measuring Tape • Place the ulnar (media/inner) border of the hand on the woman's abdomen starting from the xiphisternum (the lower end of the sternum/breastbone), and gradually proceed downwards towards the symphysis pubis lifting your hand between each step down, till you finally feel a bulge/resistance, which is the uterine fundus. Mark the level of the fundus. • Using a measuring tape, measure the distance (in cm) from the upper border of the symphysis pubis along the uterine curvature to the top of the fundus. – This is the fundal height. Note it down in the Mother and Child Protection Card – After 24 weeks of gestation, the fundal height (in cm) corresponds to the gestational age in weeks (within 1–2 cm deviation).				
Note: When measuring the fundal height, the woman's legs should be kept straight and not flexed.				

Checklist for Administrating Injection MgSO$_4$ for Initial Management of Eclampsia

S. No.	Task	Cases			
		1	2	3	4
1.	Wash hands thoroughly with soap and water and dry before and after the procedure				
2.	Keep ready 10 ampoules (20 mL = 10 g) of 50% Mg SO$_4$				
3.	Prepares 2 syringes (10 mL syringe and 22 gauze needle) with 5 g of 50% magnesium sulfate solution				
4.	Carefully cleans the injection site with an alcohol wipe.				
5.	Gives 5 g by deep IM injection in one buttock				
6.	Disposes of used needle and syringe in a puncture proof box				
7.	Carefully clean the injection site in the alternate buttock with an alcohol wipe				
8.	Give 5 g by deep IM injection into the other buttock				
9.	Dispose of used needle and syringe in puncture proof box				
10.	Record drug administered				
11.	Keep ready calcium gluconate (articulate of MgSO$_4$)				

Key Points

- If the woman is conscious, Tell her that she may experience a feeling of warmth, headache and vomiting when magnesium sulfate is given
- Refer the woman to FRU, for further necessary action. Ensure to send a referral slip with mention of 1st dose given.

Checklist for Management with Intravenous and Intramuscular Dose

S. No.	Task	Cases			
		1	2	3	4
	Administering loading dose (IV+ IM) of magnesium sulfate				
1.	Wash hands thoroughly with soap and water and air dry. Puts clean exam gloves on both hands				
2.	Prepare magnesium sulfate 20% solution, 4 g. (Take one 20 mL sterile syringe, draw 4 ampoules of Mg SO_4 (8 mL = 4 g) into the syringe, add 12 mL of distilled water/normal saline for injection to make it 20%)				
3.	Carefully clean the injection site with an alcohol wipe.				
4.	Give magnesium sulfate 20% solution, 4 g by IV injection slowly over 5 minutes				
5.	Dispose of used needle and syringe in a sharps disposal box				
	Administering IM loading dose of magnesium sulfate				
6.	Prepare 2 syringes (10 mL syringe with 22 gauze needle) with 5 g of 50% magnesium sulfate solution with 1 mL of 2% Lignocaine in the same syringe				
7.	Carefully clean the injection site with an alcohol wipe.				
8.	Give 5 g by deep IM injection in one buttock.				
9.	Dispose of used needle and syringe in a sharps disposal box				
10.	Carefully clean the injection site in the other buttock with an alcohol wipe				
11.	Give 5 g by deep IM injection into the other buttock				
12.	Dispose of used needle and syringe in a sharps disposal box				
13.	Dispose of gloves in a 0.5% decontamination solution				
14.	Washes hands thoroughly with soap and water then air dry				
15.	Record drug administration and findings on the woman's record				
	Administering IV dose of magnesium sulfate for recurrent fits/convulsions				
16.	Wash hands thoroughly with soap and water and air dry. Puts clean exam gloves on both hands.				

Contd...

Contd...

17.	Prepare syringe with 2 g magnesium sulfate (50% solution) Take one 10 mL sterile syringe, draw 2 ampoules of MgSO$_4$ 50% (4 mL = 2 g) into the syringe add 6 mL of distilled water/normal saline			
18.	Carefully clean the injection site with an alcohol wipe			
19.	Give magnesium sulfate 20% solution, 2 g by IV injection slowly over 5 minutes			
20.	Dispose of used needle and syringe in a sharps disposal box			
21.	Disposes of gloves in a 0.5% decontamination solution			
22.	Wash hands thoroughly with soap and water and dries with a clean, dry cloth or air dry.			
	Maintenance dose of MgSO$_4$			
23.	Wash hands thoroughly with soap and water and air dry. Puts clean exam gloves on both hands.			
24.	Prepare 1 syringe (10 mL syringe with 22 gauge needle) with 5 g of 50% magnesium sulfate solution with 1 mL of 2% Lignocaine in the same syringe			
25.	Carefully clean the injection site with an alcohol wipe.			
26.	Give 5 g by deep IM injection every 4 hourly in alternate buttock			
27.	Maintenance dose of MgSO$_4$ to be continued till 24 hours after delivery or the last convulsion whichever is later			
28.	Disposes of used needle and syringe in a sharps disposal box			
29.	Disposes of gloves in a 0.5% decontamination solution			
30.	Wash hands thoroughly with soap and water and dries with a clean, dry cloth or air dry			
31.	Record drug administration and findings on the woman's record			

Key Points
- If the woman is conscious, tell her that she may experience a feeling of warmth when magnesium sulfate is given
- Pregnancy induced hypertension (PIH) includes:
  - Hypertension—systolic blood pressure of 140 mm Hg or more and/or diastolic blood pressure of 90 mm Hg or more, on two consecutive readings taken four hours or more apart

- Pre-eclampsia—hypertension with proteinuria
- Eclampsia—hypertension with proteinuria and convulsions
- Always check expiry dates before using any medications
- Replenish the drug immediately after using and store at the place which is easily accessible to all staffs
- Do not give next dose of $MgSO_4$ if absent knee jerk or urinary output less than 100 mL/4 hours or respiratory rate less than 16/min
- Signs of reaction: After receiving the injection, the woman may have flushing, may feel thirsty, get a headache, feel nauseous or even vomit.
- Normal strength and availability: Magnesium Sulfate 50% w/v, 1 g in each 2 mL vial
- Keep Inj. calcium glugonate, 10%, 10 mL as an antidote.

Checklist for Management of PPH due to Retained Placenta

Situation: You are alone in a rural health facility, you gave a uterotonic medication within 1 minute of delivery, and have provided controlled cord traction during contractions and monitored your patient's bleeding for the past 30 minutes. She remains stable, but continues to bleed slowly, and her placenta has not delivered.

S. No.	Task	Cases				
		1	2	3	4	5
1.	Provide controlled cord traction with each contraction					
2.	Guard uterus while providing controlled cord traction					
3.	Identify that the placenta may be retained					
4.	Give a second dose of medication telling what dose, route and why (IV drip with Injection oxytocin 20 units in 500 ml of Ringer Lactate at 40-60 drops per minute)					
5.	Identify that the patient must be transported					
6.	The baby will be kept with the mother					
7.	Communicate respectfully and provide needed information to the mother throughout					
8.	Plan to transport mother and baby to higher centre					

Checklist for Management of PPH due to Atonic Uterus

Situation: You are alone in a rural facility. You have given 10 units of oxytocin IM and performed controlled cord traction with 3 contractions resulting in delivery of the placenta. The uterus never contracts and bleeding starts out moderate, then increases.

S. No.	Task	Cases				
		1	2	3	4	5
1.	Massage the uterus					
2.	Check the woman's bleeding					
3.	Inspect the placenta for completeness and any missing pieces					
4.	Re-check the uterus and bleeding					
5.	Give a second dose of medication telling what dose, route and why (IV drip with Injection oxytocin 20 units in 500 mL of Ringer Lactate at 40–60 drops per minute)					
6.	Re-check bleeding and tone					
	Ensure that the urinary bladder is empty					
7.	Put on long gloves					
8.	Explain to patient that you will be providing bi-manual compression					
9.	Provide bi-manual compression					
10.	Make the decision to transfer					
11.	Explain to the patient about the need to be transported for advanced care as she is at risk for complications that cannot be treated at this local facility, or is "too high risk", or "might bleed again", or may need blood transfusion					

Checklist for Abdominal Examination

S. No.	Task	Cases				
		1	2	3	4	5
1.	*Fetal lie and presentation (32 weeks onwards)*					
	Now ask the woman to flex her knees					
	a. *Carry out fundal palpation/grip* • Place both hands on the sides of the fundus to determine which part of the fetus is occupying the uterine fundus (the fetal head feels hard and globular, whereas the buttocks (breech) feel soft and irregular.					
	b. *Carry out lateral palpation/grip* • Place your hands either side of the uterus at the level of the umbilicus and apply gentle pressure. The fetal back feels like a continuous hard, flat surface on one side of the midline, while the limbs feel like irregular small knobs on the other side. • In a transverse lie, the baby's back is felt across the abdomen and the pelvic grip is empty.					
	c. *Carry out superficial pelvic grip* • Spread your right hand widely over the symphysis pubis, with the ulnar border of the hand touching the symphysis pubis. • Try to approximate the fingers and thumb, by putting gentle but deep pressure over the lower part of the uterus. The presenting part can be felt between the thumb and four fingers. Determine whether it is the head of breech (the head will feel hard and globular, and the breech soft and irregular). • If the presenting part is the head, try to move it from side to side. If it cannot be moved, it is engaged. • If neither the head, nor the buttocks are felt on the superficial pelvic grip, the baby is lying transverse. This is an abnormal lie. Refer the woman to an first referral unit (FRU) in the third trimester.					

Contd...

Contd...

	d. *Carry out deep pelvic grip (only in 3rd trimester)* • To perform this grip, face the foot end of the bed. • Place the palms of your hands on the sides of the uterus, with the fingers held close together, pointing downwards and inwards, and palpate to recognize the presenting part. • If the presenting part is the head (feels like a firm, round mass, which is ballotable, unless engaged), this maneuver, in experienced hands, will also be able to tell us about its flexion. • If the fingers diverge below the presenting part it indicates engagement of the presenting part. If the fingers converge below the presenting part it indicates that the presenting part has not engaged. • If the woman cannot relax her muscles, tell her to flex her legs slightly and to breathe deeply. Palpate in between the deep breaths. • Feel to assess if there is more than one baby.			
2.	*Fetal Heart Rate (FHR)*			
	Note: Check after 24 weeks.			
	• Place the fetoscope/bell of the stethoscope on the side of the uterus where the fetal back is felt (fetal heart sounds are best heard midway between the umbilicus and anterior superior iliac spine in the vertex and at the level of the umbilicus, or just above it in the breech). • Count the fetal heart sounds for one full minute. This is the FHR.			
	Record all your findings on the Mother and Child Protection Card and discuss them with the woman.			

Checklist for Preparation of Labor Room

S. No.	Task	Observation
1.	• Environment in the LR to be maintained with adequate lighting, cleanliness, appropriate temperature depending on the surroundings (approximately 25–28°C, curtains/screens, windows closed with intact panes, attached functional toilet with running water • Each labor table must have a light source • All the important protocols displayed at appropriate places for their reference in the labor room	
2.	Equipment needed in the LR is available and functional	
3.	Ensure that all the 7 trays are sterilized and arranged properly with labels	
4.	All the surfaces are cleaned with bleaching powder solution including the labor tables after each delivery	
5.	Arranging newborn care corner: • Radiant warmer (RW) plugged in, is functional and switched on at least half an hour before the time of delivery • A pretested and functional newborn resuscitation bag and masks are kept ready on the shelf just below the RW • A clock with seconds hand placed at prominent place.	
6.	Suction apparatus: • *For newborn*: DeeLees' suction apparatus in the tray • *For mother*: Functional foot operated/electric suction along with disposable suction catheter is available.	
7.	*Oxygen cylinder*: Check • Oxygen is available and flow is checked under water (in a bowl) before use to keep it ready for use • The knobs are pre-checked • New disposable tube is used every time oxygen is administered. • An extra full oxygen cylinder is available for back-up.	
8.	*IP practices*: • Hand washing area has soap and running water, long handle tap which can be operated with elbow • Drums to store sterilized items like gloves, instruments, linen, swabs and gauze pieces. • Exclusive functional autoclave for LR is available, delivery instruments are wrapped in a sheet and autoclaved in enough numbers (1 set for each delivery) and available as per client load autoclaving is done at least twice a day (at the end of morning and evening shift).	

Contd...

Contd...

	• Soiled instruments are first soaked in 0.5% chlorine solution before processing • PPE are used while working in the LR	
9.	*Waste disposal*: Color coded bins are available with plastic bag lining.	
10	Records: Partograph, case sheets, labor register, refer-in/refer-out registers are available and filled for each case as relevant.	

Key Points

- Temperature between 25-28°C must be maintained in LR. Hilly, cold areas will need warmers during winters
- Equipment must be checked for its functionality during change in shifts of nursing staff
- Privacy (use plastic curtains between tables) and dignity of the woman to be ensured
- Use sterilized instruments for every delivery
- LR should be draught free
- 20% buffer stock of labor room drugs must be available all the time
- NBC should not get any direct air from any corner
- Initiation of breastfeeding within one hour of childbirth
- Injection Oxytocin should be kept in fridge (not freezer)
- All the staff, doctors, nurses, cleaning staff, practice and adhere to infection prevention protocols
- The color coded bins are emptied at least once a day or as and when they get 3/4th filled.

Checklist for Kangaroo Mother Care (KMC)

S. No.	Task	Cases				
		1	2	3	4	5
1.	Counsel the mother, provides privacy to the mother. Request the mother to sit or recline comfortably					
2.	Undress the baby gently, except for cap, nappy and socks					
3.	Place the baby prone on mother's chest in an upright position with the head slightly extended, between her breasts in skin to skin contact in a frog like position; turns baby's head to one side to keep airway clear. Supports the baby's bottom with a sling/binder.					
4.	Cover the baby with mother's 'pallu' or gown; wraps the baby-mother duo with an added blanket or shawl depending upon the room temperature					
5.	Advise mother to breastfeed the baby frequently					
6.	Ensure warm room with room temperature maintained between 26–28°C					
7.	Advise the mother to provide KMC for at least 1 hour per session. The length of skin-to-skin contact should be for as long as possible					

Key Points

1. Eligibilty criteria for KMC
   - All LBW babies.
   - Sick hemodynamically stable babies needing special care(even those on IV fluid or on oxygen)
2. The two components of KMC are:
   - Skin-to-skin contact
   - Exclusive breastfeeding
3. The two prerequisites of KMC are:
   - Support to the mother in hospital and at home
   - Post-discharge follow up
4. Benefits of KMC
   - Reduces risk of hypothermia
   - Promotes lactation and weight gain
   - Reducing infections and hospital stay
   - Better bonding between mother and newborn

6
Formats

Community Survey Questionnaire

PART A: SOCIOECONOMIC AND DEMOGRAPHIC PROFILE

Name of the Respondent
Address
1. Sex:
2. Age (in completed years)
3. Religion:
4. Cast:
5. Do you have a Phone: 1. Yes.   2. No
6. Do you have a Mobile: 1. Yes.   2. No
7. Do you have transport?   1. Car   2. Jeep   3. Tractor
   4. Bullock cart   5. None
8. Education of the respondent:
   Instruction: Tick only one
   1. Illiterate
   2. Literate but no formal education
   3. School up to 5 years (Class 1-5)
   4. School up to 6-9 years (Class 6-9)
   5. Higher secondary
9. Occupation of the respondent
   Instruction: Tick only one
   1. Farmer
   2. Wage laborer
   3. Skilled worker
   4. Petty trader (shopkeeper)
   5. Self employed
   6. Under graduate
   7. Graduate/Postgraduate (general)
   8. Professional (Doctor, Engg, LLB, MBA)
   9. Technical (Diploma/IT)
   10. Others (Specify) _____

11. Service – Government
12. Service Private
13. Homemaker
15. Student
16. Retired
17. Unemployed
18. Others
10. Does the respondent's house have electricity?
    Instruction: Observe and write
    1. Yes.   2. No
11. Type of house
    Instruction: Observe and tick one
    1. Hut
    2. Semi Pucca
    3. Pucca
    4. Apartment
    5. Independent house/Bungalow
12. Where do you get your drinking water?
    Instruction: Tick only one
    1. Tap in the house
    2. Common tap
    3. Hand pump/bore well
    4. Well
    5. Tank/pond
    6. *Others*: (specify): _____
13. What type of cooking fuel do you use?
    Instruction: Tick as many as applicable
    1. LPG/Gas
    2. Kerosene
    3. Firewood
    4. Gobar gas/bio fuels
    5. Others: Specify: _____
14. What toilet arrangements do you have?
    Instruction: Tick only one
    1. Private (in your own house)
    2. Common (shared by others)
    3. Open fields
    4. Others: Specify: _____
15. Are there any persons with disabilities in the house?
    Instruction: Tick only one
    1. Yes.   2. No

16. If yes, state nature of disability:
    1. Visual
    2. Speech
17. Currently are you member of a Self Help Group?
    Instruction: Tick only one
    1. Yes.   2. No
    If yes indicate name:
    Activity:
    Is the group holding regular meeting: 1. Yes.   2. No
    Does the group have a Bank Account: 1. Yes.   2. No
18. Currently are you a member of any social group, association etc?
    Instruction: Tick only one
    1. Yes.   2. No
    If yes indicate name:
19. Indicate your economic status
    Instruction: Tick only one
    1. BPL   2. APL   3. Red Card
20. Assets owned by the Household
    Instruction: Tick as applicable
    1. Tape recorder
    2. CD player
    3. Two wheeler
    4. Electric mixer/grinder/food processor
    5. Air cooler
    6. Washing machine
    7. Car/jeep
    8. Computer
    9. Air conditioner
    10. Refrigerator
    11. Geyser
21. Name five most pressing problems faced by your community? (Indicate area and issue: e.g. health, epidemic, environment, pollution, education, drainage, roads, electricity, drinking water, sanitation, service delivery of government programs, etc.)

    Area   *Issue*
    1.
    2.
    3.
    4.
    5.

PART B: VILLAGE PROFILE

Area population:
District:
State:

1. Which of the following are there in the survey area: Provide a brief description, indicating number, type etc.
   a. Anganwadi/Play school:
   b. Primary schools:
   c. Secondary schools:
   d. Colleges:
   e. Health center (Sub centre/Primary health centre):
   f. Hospitals:
   g. Youth clubs:
   h. Sports clubs:
   i. Environment clubs:
   j. Village knowledge center/common multi media center/ common service center:
   k. Krishi Vigyan Kendra:

Family Case Study

INTRODUCTION

Community Profile

- Name of the area
- Urban/rural area
- Name of the district
- Administration
- Main caste group
- Main religion
- Occupation
- Total population

Facilities

- Medical facilities
- Health center facilities
- Education
- Social agency
- Market facilities
- Religious places
- Communication

- Community health and development program
- Post office
- Library
- Recreation facilities

Family Set Up

- Demographic profile
- Family tree
- Personal history
- Family planning immunization
- Growth and development
- Family and social relationship
- Toilet habits
- Socioeconomic background
- Floor map
- Furniture
- Storage of water and food
- Washing places
- Bathing areas
- Latrines
- Surroundings
- Family health attitudes, beliefs and practices
  - Disease
  - Cause and spread
  - Food
  - Immunization

Physical Examination

- Anthropometric measurement
- Vital signs
- Head-to-foot assessment

GROWTH AND DEVELOPMENT

Nutritional Assessment

- Anthropometric assessment
- Bio-medical assessment, e.g. blood, stool and urine examination
- Clinical examination, e.g. alopecia, pyorrhea
- 24 hours recall

Time	Foodstuff	Amount

Time	Foodstuff	Amount	Cooked volume	Uncooked volume	Protein	Fat	Calcium	Iron	kcal

- Comparison of client and recommended value

Content	Client value	Recommended value	Remarks

- Modified diet plan

Time	Foodstuff	Amount	Cooked volume	Uncooked volume	Protein	Fat	Calcium	Iron	kcal

Nursing Process
- Individual
- Family
- Community

Theory Application

Home Visit

General information
- Name
- Age
- Sex
- Classification

Problems	Needs

Short-term goal	Long-term goal

Knowledge, Attitude and Practice (KAP)

Pre-teaching	Post-teaching

Health Education

Specific objective	Content	Teaching-learning activity	Audio-visual aids	Evaluation

Records of Procedure

S. No.	Date	Procedure done	Remarks	Signature

SUMMARY

Self Evaluation

Conclusion

Review of Literature
- Journal abstract
- WHO report
- Epidemiological study.

BIBLIOGRAPHY

Books

Author's last name, first name. *Book title.* Additional information. City of publication: Publishing company, publication date.

Encyclopedia and Dictionary

Author's last name, first name. "Title of Article." *Title of Encyclopedia.* Date.

Magazine and Newspaper Articles

Author's last name, first name. "Article title." *Periodical title* Volume # Date: inclusive pages.

Website or Webpage

Author's last name, first name (if available). "Title of work within a project or database." *Title of site, project, or database.* Editor (if available). Electronic publication information (Date of publication or of the latest update, and name of any sponsoring institution or organization). Date of access and <full URL>.

School Health Record

1. Name:
2. Class:
3. DOB:
4. Father's name:
5. Address:
6. School name:
7. Income:

Parent's Signature   **Principal Signature**

With seal.

S. No.	Class	1st visit	2nd visit	3rd visit	4th visit	5th visit	6th visit	7th visit	8th visit	9th visit	10th visit
	Weight										
	Height										
1.	Protein-energy malnutrition										
2.	HB										
3.	Vitamin deficiency										
4.	Skin										
5.	Vision										
6.	Dental caries										

Contd...

Contd...

S. No.	Class	1st visit	2nd visit	3rd visit	4th visit	5th visit	6th visit	7th visit	8th visit	9th visit	10th visit
7.	ENT										
8.	Warm infestation										
9.	Cardiac diseases										
10.	Joint pain										
11	Convulsion										
12.	Mental illness										
13.	Others										

Physician Signature

Date	Problems encountered	Treatment given	Reference	Physician signature

7 Procedure

Vaginal Examination

CHECKLIST FOR VAGINAL EXAMINATION DURING FIRST STAGE OF LABOR

S. No.	Task	Cases			
		1	2	3	4
1.	Wash the hands properly before and after each vaginal examination.				
2.	Wear plastic apron and surgical gloves				
3.	Explain the woman about the procedure and always take consent before doing it.				
4.	Clean perineum with diluted savlon swab, discard the soiled swab in red container				
5.	Use middle and index finger of right/left hand and insert them into vagina at 12' O Clock -6' O clock position				
6.	Judges the dilatation of cervix-in cms				
7.	Assess the adequacy of the pelvis by noting well curved sacrum and inability to reach both ischial spines at the same time				
8.	Remove gloves and puts them into 0.5% chlorine solution				
9.	Inform the woman about the progress of labor				
10.	Record the information on the partograph, if cervical dilatation is 4 cm and above				

Key Points
- Do per vaginal (P/V) examination only when required/indicated to minimize the infection
- Maintain privacy and dignity of women at all times

BP Recording

CHECKLIST FOR BLOOD PRESSURE (BP) RECORDING

S. No	Task	Cases			
		1	2	3	4
1.	Check that bulb is properly attached to the tubing				
2.	Check for any crack and leakage in the bulb and cuff				
3.	Check mercury column knob is in open mode				
4.	Ask the person to sit on a chair or lie down on flat surface				
5.	Place the apparatus on a horizontal surface at the person's heart level				
6.	The mercury column is at the observer's eye level.				
7.	Ties the cuff 1 inch above the elbow placing both the tubes in front				
8.	Raise the pressure of the cuff to 30 mm Hg above the level at which pulse is no longer felt				
9.	Release pressure slowly and listens with stethoscope keeping it on brachial artery at the elbow				
10.	Note the reading where the sound is heard (systolic pressure)				
11.	Follow the sound and note reading where the sound disappears (diastolic)				
12.	Deflate and remove the cuff; closes the mercury column knob				
13.	Record the reading on MCP card				

Key Points BP Recording

- In a pregnant woman, BP must be recorded during each visit.
- Hypertension is diagnosed when two consecutive readings taken 4 hours or more apart show the systolic blood pressure to be 140 mm Hg or more and/or the diastolic blood pressure to be 90 mm Hg or more.
- High blood pressure during pregnancy may signify pregnancy-induced hypertension (PIH) and/or chronic hypertension.

- If the woman has high blood pressure, check her urine for the presence of albumin. The presence of albumin (+2) together with high blood pressure is sufficient to categorise her as having pre-eclampsia. Refer her to the medical officer (MO) immediately.
- If the diastolic blood pressure of the woman is above 110 mm Hg, it is a danger sign that points towards imminent eclampsia. The urine albumin should be estimated at the earliest. If it is strongly positive, the woman should be referred to the first referral unit (FRU) immediately.
- If the woman has high blood pressure but no urine albumin, she should be referred to the MO at 24 hours primary health center (PHC).
- A woman with PIH, pre-eclampsia or imminent eclampsia requires hospitalisation and supervised treatment at a 24-hour PHC/FRU.
- Reading must be entered in the Medical card.

Hb Estimation

CHECKLIST FOR HEMOGLOBIN ESTIMATION

S. No.	Task	Cases			
		1	2	3	4
1.	Keep all the necessary items ready (Sahli's Hb meter, N/10 HCl, gloves, spirit swabs, lancet, distill water and dropper, puncture proof container, 0.5% chlorine solution)				
2.	Wash hands and wear gloves				
3.	Clean the Hb tube and pipette				
4.	Fill the HB tube with 0.1 N HCl with the dropper				
5.	Clean tip of the person's ring finger with spirit swab				
6.	Prick the finger with lancet and discards first drop of blood				
7.	Allow a large blood drop to form on the finger tip and sucks it with pipette upto 20 cmm mark. Take care that air entry is prevented while sucking the blood				
8.	Wipe tip of the pipette and transfer the blood to the Hb tube containing N/10 HCl				

Contd...

Contd...

S. No.	Task	Cases			
		1	2	3	4
9.	Rinse the pipette 2–3 times with N/10 HCl				
10.	Leave the solution in test tube for 10 minutes				
11.	After 10 minutes, dilutes the acid by adding distil water drop-by-drop and mix it with stirrer				
12.	Match with the color of the comparator				
13.	Note down the reading (lower meniscus)				
14.	Dispose off the used lancet in puncture proof container				
15.	Drop the used gloves in 0.5% chlorine solution				

Key Points-Hb Estimation

- In a pregnant woman, Hb estimation must be done during each visit.
- The initial hemoglobin level will serve as a baseline with which the later results, obtained at the three subsequent antenatal visits, can be compared.
- Interpretation of findings:
    - Hb > 11 g% (absence of anemia)-
        - Prophylactic iron folic acid (IFA) tablet (100 mg elemental iron and 0.5 mg folic acid) once a day for 100 days
        - Starting after the first trimester, at 14–16 weeks of gestation
        - Regimen is to be repeated for three months post-partum.
    - Hb 7–11 g% (moderate anemia)-
        - Therapeutic IFA tablet twice a day.
        - Regimen is to be repeated for 3 months postpartum.
    - Hb < 7 g% (severe anemia) or those who have breathlessness and tachycardia (pulse rate of more than 100 beats per minute) due to anemia-
        - Start the therapeutic dose of IFA and
        - Refer the woman to FRU.

Urine Testing for Protein and Sugar

CHECKLIST FOR URINE TESTING

S. No.	Task	Observations
1.	Keep all the necessary items ready (urine specimen collection bottles/container and dipsticks, red bin)	
2.	Check the expiry date on the kit	
3.	Remove one strip from the bottle and replace the cap	
4.	Completely immerse reagent area of the strip in the urine and remove it immediately	
5.	While removing the strip from urine run the edge against the rim of the container to wipe off the excess urine	
6.	For glucose: After 30 seconds compare the blue colored reagent area against the color chart area on the bottle and records the finding	
7.	For protein: After 60 seconds compare the yellow colored reagent area against the color chart area on the bottle and records the finding	
8.	Discard the stick in red bin.	

Key Points-Urine Test

- In a pregnant woman, urine testing for protein and sugar must be done during each visit.
- *Testing the urine for the presence of protein (albumin)* is a very important test used for the detection of pre-eclampsia, which (along with eclampsia) is one of the five major causes of maternal mortality.
- *Testing urine for the presence of sugar* is a test used to diagnose women with gestational diabetes (which may cause delivery-related complications due to the infant's large size, development of diabetes later in life, increased risk of newborn death and stillbirth or low blood sugar (glucose) or illness in the newborn, and *jaundice*)
- The presence of albumin together with high blood pressure is sufficient to categorize her as having pre-eclampsia. Refer her to the MO immediately
- If urine is positive for sugar, refer her to the MO to get her blood sugar examined and a glucose tolerance test carried out, if required
- Reading must be entered in the Medical card
- Store the tightly sealed bottle in cool dark place
- Each strip should be used only once.

Bag Technique

The *bag technique* is a tool by which the nurse, during her visit will enable her to perform a nursing procedure with ease and deftness, to save time and effort with the end view of rendering effective nursing care to clients.

The *public health bag* is an essential and indispensable equipment of a public health nurse which she has to carry along during her home visits. It contains basic medication and articles which are necessary for giving care.

Principles

- Performing the bag technique will minimize, if not, prevent the spread of any infection.
- It saves time and effort in the performance of nursing procedures.
- The bag technique can be performed in a variety of ways depending on the agency's policy, the home situation, or as long as principles of avoiding transfer of infection is always observed.

Contents of the Bag

- Paper lining
- Extra paper for making bag for waste materials (paper bag)

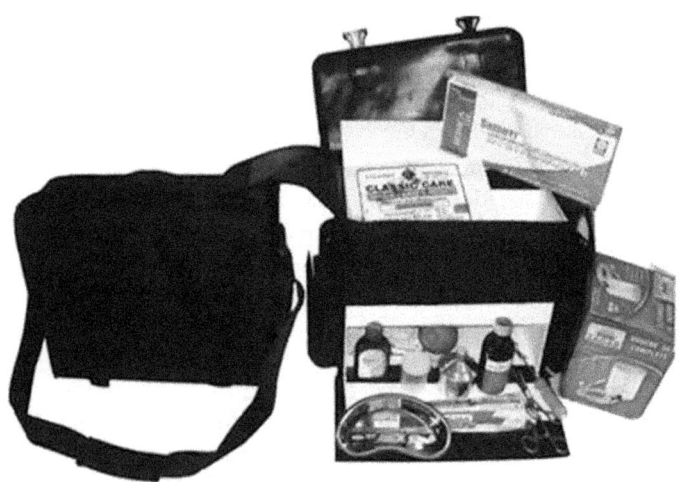

Fig.1: Community bag with articles.

- Plastic linen/lining
- Apron
- Hand towel in plastic bag
- Soap in soap dish
- Thermometers
- 2 pairs of scissors [1 surgical and 1 bandage]
- 2 pairs of forceps [curved and straight]
- Syringes [5 mL and 2 mL]
- Hypodermic needles g. 19, 22, 23, 25
- Sterile dressings
- Sterile cord tie
- Adhesive plaster
- Dressing [OS, cotton ball]
- Tape measure
- Baby's scale
- 1 pair of gloves
- 2 test tubes
- Test tube holder
- Medicines
  - Betadine
  - Ophthalmic ointment (antibiotic)
  - Hydrogen peroxide
  - Spirit
  - Acetic acid
  - Benedict's solution

Note: *Blood pressure apparatus and stethoscope are carried separately.*

Steps/Procedures

Actions	Rationale
1. Upon arriving at the client's home, place the bag on the table or any flat surface lined with paper lining, clean side out (folded part touching the table). Put the bag's handles or strap beneath the bag.	To protect the bag from contamination.
2. Ask for a basin of water and a glass of water if faucet is not available. Place these outside the work area.	To be used for hand washing. To protect the work field from being wet.
3. Open the bag, take the linen/plastic lining and spread over work field or area. The paper lining, clean side out (folded part out).	To make a non-contaminated work field or area.

Contd...

Contd...

Actions	Rationale
4. Take out hand towel, soap dish and apron and place them at one corner of the work area (within the confines of the linen/plastic lining).	To prepare for hand washing.
5. Do hand washing. Wipe, dry with towel. Leave the plastic wrappers of the towel in a soap dish in the bag.	Hand washing prevents possible infection from one care provider to the client.
6. Put on apron right side out and wrong side with crease touching the body, sliding the head into the neck strap. Neatly tie the straps at the back.	To protect the nurses' uniform. Keeping the crease creates aesthetic appearance.
7. Put out things most needed for the specific case (e.g.) thermometer, kidney basin, cotton ball, waste paper bag) and place at one corner of the work area.	To make them readily accessible.
8. Place waste paper bag outside of work area.	To prevent contamination of clean area.
9. Close the bag.	To give comfort and security, maintain personal hygiene and hasten recovery.
10. Proceed to the specific nursing care or treatment.	To prevent contamination of bag and contents.
11. After completing nursing care or treatment, clean and alcoholize the things used.	To protect caregiver and prevent spread of infection to others.
12. Do hand washing again.	
13. Open the bag and put back all articles in their proper places.	
14. Remove apron folding away from the body, with soiled side folded inwards, and the clean side out. Place it in the bag.	
15. Fold the linen/plastic lining, clean; place it in the bag and close the bag.	
16. Make post-visit conference on matters relevant to health care, taking anecdotal notes preparatory to final reporting.	To be used as reference for future visit.
17. Make appointment for the next visit, taking note of the date, time and purpose.	For follow-up care.

After Care
1. Before keeping all articles in the bag, clean and alcoholize them.
2. Get the bag from the table, fold the paper lining (and insert), and place in between the flaps and cover the bag.

Evaluation and Documentation
3. Record all relevant findings about the client and members of the family.
4. Take note of environmental factors which affect the clients/family health.
5. Include quality of nurse-patient relationship.
6. Assess effectiveness of nursing care provided.

Dementia Scale

BLESSED DEMENTIA SCALE
Name of the client:
Students name:
Date:

Instruction: One point for each correct answer Score

CHANGES IN PERFORMANCE OF EVERYDAY ACTIVITIES
- Inability to perform household tasks
- Inability to cope with small sums of money
- Inability to remember shortlist of items
- Inability to find way about indoor
- Inability to find way about familiar streets
- Inability to interpret surroundings (e.g. whether in hospital or home)
- Inability to recall recent events (e.g. visit of relatives or friends)
- Tendency to dwell in the past.

CHANGES IN HABITS
Eating
(0) = Cleanly, with proper utensils
(1) = Messily, with spoon only
(2) = Simple solids, e.g. biscuits
(3) = Has to be fed

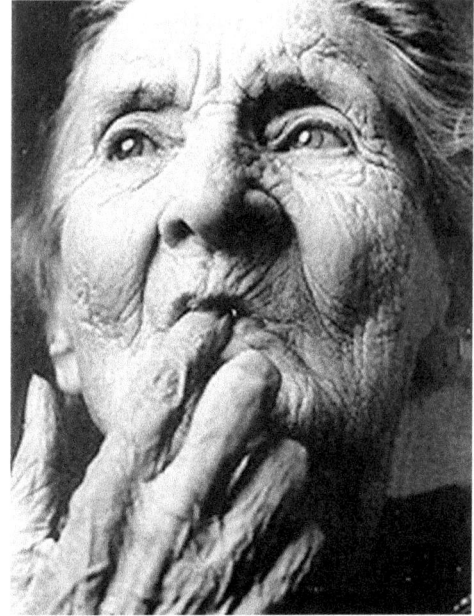

Fig. 2: Alzheimer's disease.

Dressing

(0) = Unaided
(1) = Occasionally misplaced buttons, etc
(2) = Wrong sequence, commonly forgetting items

Sphincter Control

(0) = Complete control
(1) = Occasionally wet bed
(2) = Doubly incontinent

CHANGES IN PERSONALITY, INTEREST, DRIVE

- Increased rigidity
- Increased egocentricity
- Impairment of regard of feeling for others
- Coarsening of affect
- Impairment of emotional control
- Hilarity in inappropriate situations

- Diminished emotional responsiveness
- Sexual misdemeanor
- Hobbies relenquised
- Diminished initiative or growing apathy
- Purposeless hyperactivity

Results

- Mild dementia (Score: 0–5)
- Moderate dementia (Score: 6–11)
- Severe dementia (Score: 12–17)

Mini Mental Status Examination

S. No.	Questions	Maximum score	Obtained score
1.	Orientation i. What is the (year), (season), (date), (day) and (month)? ii. Where are we (state), (country), (town), (area) and (street)	5 5	
2.	Registration Name three objects and ask them to repeat?	3	
3.	Attention Serials 7 substraction starting from 100	5	
4.	Recall Ask for the three object repeated above?	3	
5.	Language 1. Name a pencil and watch? 2. Repeat the following 3. Follow command 4. Write a sentence 5. Copy the design shown	2 1 3 1 1	

Total score   20

Inference:

8

Strategies to Control Emerging Diseases

INTRODUCTION

The World Health Report shows that the world stands on the brink of a global crisis in infectious diseases. No country is safe from them and no country can afford to ignore their threat any longer. Today the infectious diseases are not only a health issue, they have become a social problem with tremendous consequences for the well being of the individual and and community. According to the National Health Policy (NHP) of India 2002, the major health problems are infectious diseases. These diseases can be prevented by health personnel such as nurses. Some infectious diseases once thought to be all but conquered have returned with the vengeance. Others have developed stubborn resistance to antibiotic drugs new and previously unknown diseases continue to emerge. Together, these trends amount to a crisis for today and a challenging for the future. In 1997, the theme chosen by the WHO to celebrate the World Health Day was "Emerging Infectious Diseases: Global Alert-Global Response". That was as a wake-up call for the member countries to develop strategies to meet the challenges in combating emerging infectious diseases.

The factor responsible for emergence and re-emergence of infectious disease are:
- Unplanned and under planned urbanization
- Overcrowding and rapid population growth
- Poor sanitation
- Inadequate public health infrastructure
- Resistance to antibiotics
- Increased exposure of humans to disease vectors and reservoirs of infection in nature
- Rapid and intense international travel.

Effect of deforestation and use of land for cultivation and/or human settlement. As settlers come in contact with vectors and are exposed to large number of new viral, parasitic, and bacterial disease agents. In India, for example, people going to forest to collect wood were bitten by ticks and came down with Kyasanur forest disease. Malaria has spread along the irrigation canal in the desert areas of Rajasthan in India,

Chapter 8 Strategies to Control Emerging Diseases

likewise the laying of Konkan Railway lines has carried the malaria vector in areas where malaria did not exist Effect of drought followed by heavy rains Global warming and its effect on span of life-cycle.

Strategies

- Understanding environmental factors which facilitate emergence, maintenance and transmission of these disease
- Studying the evaluation of pathogenic infectious agents resulting in changes in infectivity, virulence transmissibility and adaptations
- Knowing host factors influencing emergence of new infection and their transmission
- Development of tools for diagnosis, management, control and prophylaxis
- Training and infrastructure for responding to emerging disease
- Information sharing on emerging infections
- Development of research-based evidence to influence policy modifications
- Isolation
- Hand washing
- Dust control
- Disinfection
- Control of droplet infection
- Administrative measures
- There should be a "Control of Infection Committee" to formulate policies regarding admission of infectious cases. Isolation facilitates disinfection procedures, etc.
- Improved training for scientists, clinicians, public health professionals who can be mobilized to respond to these threats
- Availability of laboratory with adequate bio-safety levels
- Training of staff to work in high/maximum, containment laboratories.
- Stable financial support
- Establishing and strengthening surveillance system for infectious diseases. Surveillance indicates where a disease has suddenly appeared and gives vital clues about how the emergent infectious agent may spread
- Development of new field-applicable diagnostic tests to facilitate surveillance
- Research on biomedical applications of new technology such as remote sensing, Geographical Information System (GIS) to improve ability to predict future infectious disease outbreaks.
- Development of vaccines to block the transmission of microbial pathogens, genetic alteration of a vector to prevent a pathogen from replicating within it

- Detecting and limiting environmental sources of contamination, such as water supplies. Validate current epidemiologic and modeling studies to assess the effectiveness of control methods in regions where drug resistance is a problem development of models to demonstrate the impact of delays in implementing outbreak control measures and increasing the number of index cases on the incidence of cases of simulated outbreaks
- Networks need to be developed between various agencies and institutions involved in research in emerging infections to share their experiences, data and concerns. A regional network of networks would help tremendously in sharing of information.

H1 N1 Flu

- Strategy for India
  - Treatment with antiviral drugs (vaccine is at present not available anywhere in the world)
- Blood sample
  - 2 weeks later another sample by the method of raising antibody titer.
  - Health Department would send teams to monitor them at home, unless this is done chances are that the virus will be transmitted within the community and spread fast.
  - The Director of Public health would also provide prophylactic doses of Tamiflu for prevention to close relatives of those who have A (H1 N1) flu
  - Additionally staff at all the hospitals identified to quarantine patients would be trained in lifting samples and preparing them for dispatch to the Institute of Communicable Disease, Delhi.
  - The Director General of Health Services (Emergency Medical Relief) has recognized three laboratories in Tamil Nadu as test been centers for A H1 N1 flu.
  - The three labs are King Institute of Preventive Medicine, Guindy.
  - Christian Medical College, Vellore
  - JIPMER, Puducherry.
  - The National Institute of Communicable Diseases, New Delhi, and the National Institute of Virology will remain the apex centers to guide the labs and verify results.
  - Apart from these two institutes and the three institutes in Chennai, 13 other established laboratories have been recognized to test for A (H1 N1). In addition to handling the cases within the State, they will also help out neighboring States that do not have such labs, thereby covering the entire country.

Chapter 8 Strategies to Control Emerging Diseases

Innovative NRHM Schemes

- The Union Health and Family Welfare Ministry has recommended an in-depth review of 20 innovative schemes being implemented by states and Union Territories under the NRHM for scaling up and replication
- The term innovative has been used flexibly under the NRHM and encompasses pilot projects
- Creative use of public private partnerships across a range of services
- Use of cash transfers and demand side financial mechanism to give better outcomes
- And also to address equity issues
- The NRHM which focuses on decentralized planning, implementation and flexibility to states and the implementation agencies has resulted is a number of innovations with impressive results
- The innovations identified are:
  - Chiranjeevi Yojana (Gujarat)
  - Delivery Huts (Haryana)
  - Rural Emergency Health Transportation scheme
  - Scheme (Andhra Pradesh)
  - Mobile Health Clinic (West Bengal)
  - Mobile Boat Clinic in Riverine Area (Assam)
  - Subcontracting out of diagnostic services in rural area.
  - Security scavenging and waste management and mechanized laundry services as done by West Bengal.
- Management of PHCs by NGO's in Arunachal Pradesh.
- Communitarian private public partnership for management of health centres
- Rapid diffusion of IUCD Training Programme using Alternate Training methology is 12 states, including, TN CA MT (Center for Advanced Midwifery Training)
- Family counseling centers (Madhya Pradesh, Rajasthan, Odisha, Maharashtra, Kerala)
- The NHP (National Health Programme) 2002 states that public health delivery Center's need to make a beginning by increasing the number of nursing personnel. Therefore, to overcome the shortages and as per NHP 2002 plans, there is a need to modify nursing staffing norms to provide essential health interventions to the community health nursing services at various levels.

Strategy for Meeting the Challenges in Nursing for the Delivery of Health Intervention
- Strengthen involvement of nurses in health and nursing policy formulation and planning.
- Empower nurse leaders.
- Establish a quality assurance system for the nursing service is the community.
- Ensure nursing workforce management as an integral part of human resource planning and health system development.
- Enhance nursing autonomy is practice.
- Enforce implementation of recommended norms on nurse to client ratio.
- Create post for professional nurses at the community level and produce advanced practice nurses.
- Ensure appropriate facilities and adequate medical equipment and supplies.
- Promote evidence-based practice and nursing research.
- Establish a continuing nursing education system.
- Strengthen payment scales, incentive systems and working conditions.
- Ensure quality of nursing education by strengthening nursing programmes, increasing qualified nurse educators and allocating appropriate resources to maximize efficiency and effectiveness.
- Expand the role and authority of the Indian Nursing Council on Nursing Development by revision of the Act, Restructuring and networking.
- Strengthen the competency of the auxiliary nurse-midwife.

Infrastructure Required at Various Levels of the Health Care Services
- Sub-centre population 5,000
  - To be manned by 2 year's trained staff as per the revised syllabus
  - Male health worker and one public health nurse
  - Strengthening the infrastructural facilities.
- PHC 30,0000 Population
  - One PHN practitioner (with additional training) and one PHN supervisor to effectively supervise all Maternal child health services and family welfare services
  - 4 Staff nurses for 24 hours service
- CHC one lakh Population
  - 14 staff nurses
  - 3 PHN supervisors

Chapter 8 Strategies to Control Emerging Diseases

- 1 PHN Practitioner
- 1 Independent midwifery practitioner
- District level
  - Strengthen the institution of the DPHN officer to supervise and monitor the Nursing and midwifery system
  - 2 PHN officers

Keys to Good Health

- Hygiene and sanitation
- Family planning
- *Safe motherhood*: Antenatal period
- Nutrition of children
- Immunization of babies
- Managing common illnesses

CONCLUSION

Community Health Nurses can make major contributions to health care development and achieve the Millennium Development Goals only if there is strong support at the policy level to ensure policy implementation. Strong commitment and close collaboration between professional organizations, nursing services institutes are needed in planning, implementation and evaluation of nursing workforce management. Maximal use of resources within the country is essential. Best practices from each State need to be shared, learned and recognized. In addition community health nurses should commit themselves to continuously improve the quality of nursing services by strengthening their competencies.

9 Miscellaneous

Invention	Year	Inventor	Nation
Antibiotic	1928	Prof Alexander Fleming	Britain
Artificial limbs	16th century	Ambrose pare	France
Ayurveda	2000-1000BC	Atreya	India
Bacteria	1683	Leewenhock	Netherland
Bacteriology	1872	Ferdinand cohn	Germany
BP Machine	1896	Dr Scipione Riva Rocci	Italy
Hearing aid	1902	King Edward vil	Britain
Insulin	1921	Frederick and Charlest best banting	Canada and Britain
Siddha,Yoga	C 750 AD	Vrudukunta	India
Smallpox eradicate	1980	WHO Declaration	
Stethoscope	1819	Rene Laenec	France
Thermometer	1592	Edward Calvin	USA
Vaccination	1796	Edward Jenner	London
Vitamin	1912	Sir FJ Hopkins	Britain
Vit-A	1913	Mccollum and M Davis	USA
Vit-B1	1936	Minot and Murphy	USA
Vit-C	1919	Frolich Holst	Norway
Vit-D	1925	Mecollum	USA
Yoga	200-100BC	Patanjali	India
APGAR	1952	Virginia Apgar	

DO YOU KNOW THAT

- Betin is a powerful cancer inhibitor
- Groundnut oil can strengthen the urinary bladder
- Capsicum can help cure uterine disorder

- Leaves of custard apple can cure skin eczema and ulcers
- Chikhu can cure arthritis
- Applying milk cream on raw wounds can arrest bleeding
- Hookworm abundance is the prime cause of anemia in children
- Skin and bones heal by taking sea foods, watermelon, black gram.

MEDICAL ABBREVIATION

- Ab–Antibody
- Acc–Accident
- Af–Afebrile
- Alc–Alcohol
- Aq–Water
- ARI–Acute respiratory tract infection
- BCG–Bacillus Calmette-Guerin vaccine
- BR–Bed Rest
- BW–Birth weight
- Ca–Calcium
- Cho–Carbohydrate
- Comm–Communicable
- *E. coli*–*Escherichia coli*
- FA–First aid
- Fe def–Iron deficiency
- FHR–Fetal heart rate
- FTND–Full term normal delivery
- g–Gram
- H/A–Headache
- Hb–Hemoglobin
- HIV–Human immunodeficiency virus
- Ht–Height
- IUD–Intrauterine device
- IUCP–Intrauterine contraceptive device
- IUGR–Intrauterine growth retardation
- LBW–Low birth weight
- NB–Newborn
- Nullipara–Never gave birth
- AEFI–Adverce effect of even following immunization
- NVD–Nausea, vomiting, diarrhea
- TPR–Temperature, pulse, respiration
- T_x–Treatment
- URI–Upper respiratory infection
- Yrs–Years

NURSING EMERGENCY KIT

A nursing kit for emergencies has been designed keeping in mind the various activities to be undertaken by the nurse.

- Dressing materials
- First aid
- Oral rehydration salts (ORS) packet
- Iron folic acid (IFA) tablets
- DD kits
- Contraceptives
- Chloroscope
- Urine testing kit
- Hand washing articles
- Chlorine tablets
- Medicines for minor ailments
- Stationary
- Family health card
- Gen health quest for screening for mental health problems.

Index

Page numbers followed by f refer to figure, and t refer to table

A

Abdominal examination 83
 checklist for 91
Accredited Social Health Activist 67
Acid indigestion 56
Adult assessment 15
Albumin 109
Alzheimer's disease 114f
Animal bite 62
Antenatal assessment 21f
Antenatal examination 20
Antenatal history 23
 format 17
Anthropometric measurement 1, 4, 7, 10, 13, 16
Ascorbic acid 45, 46
Atonic uterus 90

B

Baby resuscitation equipment 70
Baby's breathing 76
Bacillus Calmette-Guerin 5
Back pain 62
Bag
 contents of 110
 technique 110
Balanced diet 38, 39, 47t, 48t
Blessed dementia scale 113
Blood pressure
 apparatus 111
 recording 106
  checklist for 106
  key points 106
Body weight 45, 46
Breastfeeding, checklist for 78
Burns 59
 home remedies for 59f

C

Calcium 45, 46
Calories 51
Carbohydrate 41, 47
Center for Advanced Midwifery Training 119
Chiranjeevi yojana 119
Cold 60
 compress at home 58f
Common animal bites 62f
Communication 32
Community
 bag with articles 110f
 nutrition 37
 profile 99
 survey questionnaire 96
Conjunctivitis 63
Constipation 56
 home remedies of 57f
Control emerging diseases 116
Controlled cord traction 73
Convulsions 86, 88
Coughs 58
Counseling, preparation for 79

D

Deep pelvic grip 92
Delivery, conduction of 71
Dementia scale 113
Demographic profile 17
Developmental milestones 4, 7, 9, 12
Diagnostic services in rural area, subcontracting out of 119
Diarrhea 55
 signs of 56f
 symptoms of 56f
Dietary reference intakes 38
Dietary supplements 38
Dressing 114

E

Eating 113
Eclampsia 88
 initial management of 85
Emerging infectious diseases 116
Energy 40, 47
Essential newborn care 69, 72

F

Family case study 99
Family planning counseling 80
 checklist on 79
Family set up 100
Fat 40, 45-47, 53
Feeding reflexes 2
Fetal
 heart rate 92
 lie and presentation 91
 surface 75
Fever 57
First referral unit 107
Five food group 40*t*
 system 39
Fluids 31
Folic acid 45, 46
Food
 availability of 42
 composition database 40
 exchange lists 39
 functional 38
 group 40, 47, 48
 health value of 42
 labeling and surveillance
   system 39
 list 44
 supplements 38
Fundal palpation/grip 91

G

General counseling skills 79
Geographical information
   system 117
Gestational age
 correct estimation of 83
 estimation, checklist for 83
Glucose 109
Gomez classification 16

Growth
 and development 100
 promotion and monitoring 10

H

H1 N1 118
Head
 lice 61
 delivery of 71
 to foot
  assessment 5, 7, 11, 14, 16
  examination 20, 24
Headaches 58
Health
 care services 120
 education 102
Healthy diet 51
Hemoglobin estimation 107
 checklist for 107
 key points 108
Hepatitis B 5
Household cures 55
Hypertension 88
 chronic 106
 pregnancy-induced 87, 106
Hyperthermia 68

I

Immunization 5, 8, 11, 14
Inactivated polio vaccine 5
Infant physical assessment 3, 4*f*
Infection
 prevention equipment and
   supplies 70
 risk for 66
Insect bites and stings 61
Intramuscular dose, checklist for
   management with 86
Intranatal assessment format 22
Intrauterine contraceptive device,
   postpartum 70
Intravenous dose, checklist for
   management with 86
Iron 45, 46

J

Japanese encephalitis 6
Jaundice 109

Index **127**

K

Kangaroo mother care, checklist for 95
Knowledge, attitude and practice 102

L

Labor
 first stage of 105
 room, checklist for preparation of 93
 second stage of 69
 third stage of 69, 72, 73
Lateral palpation/grip 91
Literature, review of 102
Lower vagina, examination of 74

M

Magazine and newspaper articles 102
Magnesium sulphate
 administering injection 85
 intramuscular loading dose of 86
 intravenous loading dose of 86
 loading dose of 86
 maintenance dose of 87
Main nutrients 40
Malnutrition, severe acute 10
Meal plan 42
Measles 6
Membranes 75
 examination of 74
Mental
 health 35
 status 24
Menu plan 37
 portion size for 47*t*
Mid-upper arm circumference
 interpretation of 10, 13
 screening 13*f*
 advantages of 10, 14
 tape 10*f*
Mini mental status examination 115
Minor ailments 55
Minor cut
 and grazes 61
 management 61*f*

Mobile Boat Clinic in Riverine Area 119
Mobile Health Clinic 119
Moderate Acute Malnutrition 10
Mother after delivery, immediate care of 76

N

National Health Policy 116
National Health Programme 119
National Institute of Communicable Diseases 118
National Institute of Nutrition 41
National Institute of Virology 118
Net energy 45, 46
Newborn resuscitation, checklist for 77
Nicotinic acid 45, 46
Non-communicable diseases 51, 52
Normal delivery 69
Nose bleeding 60
 care of 60*f*
Nurse, role of 3, 6, 8, 12, 15
Nursing care 2, 6, 8, 11, 15, 17, 30
 in community, steps of 65*f*
Nursing emergency kit 124
Nutrition 19, 32
Nutritional assessment 100
 and screenings, tool for 39
Nutritional counselling, tool for 39
Nutritional status, assessment of 16

O

Oral poliovirus vaccines 5
Oxygen
 adequacy of 32
 cylinder 93

P

Pain 34
 scale 62*f*
Partner's health history 20
Pentavalent 5
Per vaginal examination findings 25
Perineum, examination of 74
Phytochemicals 38
Placenta, examination of 74

Planning diets 41
   principles of 41
Postnatal assessment 26
Postnatal care 26*f*
Postpartum hemorrhage, checklist for management of 89, 90
Potassium 53
Pre-eclampsia 88
Pre-schooler assessment 9
Primary Health Center 56, 107
Protective reflexes 2
Protein 45, 46, 47
   energy malnutrition assessment
      children 10, 13
      infant 10
   testing urine for presence of 109
   urine testing for 109
Proteinuria 88
Public health bag 110
Pyridoxine 45, 46

R

Recommended dietary allowances 38, 44, 45*t*
Recurrent fits 86
Reflexes 2
Respiratory infection 59*f*
Resuscitation, newborn 76
Riboflavin 45, 46
Rotaviruse 5
Rural community, assessment in 18*f*
Rural Emergency Health Transportation Scheme 119

S

Salt 53
   sugar solution 58
School going assessment 12
School health record 103
Shoulders, delivery of 71
Simple vomiting, control of 57
Socialization 35
Socioeconomic and demographic profile 96
Sodium 53
Sphincter control 114
Sprain 60
   management 60*f*
Stethoscope 111
Stomach ulcers 56
Suction apparatus 93
Sugar 54
   testing urine for presence of 109
   urine testing for 109
Superficial pelvic grip 91
Systematic assessment 5, 8, 11, 14, 17

T

Theory application 101
Thiamine 45, 46
Toddler assessment 7
Tolerable upper intake level 38

U

Umbilical cord 75
   examination of 74
Urine test
   checklist for 109
   key points 109
Uterine massage 74

V

Vaginal examination 105
   checklist for 105
Various age groups, assessment of 1
Ventilation, assess state of 32
Village profile 99
Vital signs 1, 7, 10, 14, 16, 24
Vitamin
   A 6, 45, 46
   B12 45, 46
Vomiting 55

W

Waste, decontamination and disposal of 75
World Health Day 116
World Health Report 116

EU GSPR Authorised Reprsentative
Logos Europe, 9 rue Nicolas Poussin
1700, La Rochelle, France
Phone: +33 (0) 6 67 93 73 78
E-mail: contact@logoseurope.eu